Multicultural Human Services for AIDS Treatment and Prevention:
Policy, Perspectives, and Planning

Multicultural Human Services for AIDS Treatment and Prevention: Policy, Perspectives, and Planning

Julio Morales, PhD
Marcia Bok, PhD
Editors

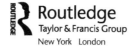

Routledge
Taylor & Francis Group
New York London

First published by The Haworth Press, Inc.

This edition published 2013 by Routledge
711 Third Avenue, New York, NY 10017
2 Park Square, Milton Park, Abingdon, Oxon, OX14 4RN

Routledge is an imprint of the Taylor & Francis Group, an informa business

Multicultural Human Services/or AIDS Treatment and Prevention: Policy, Perspectives, and Planning has also been published as *Journal of Multicultural Social Work,* Volume 2, Number 3 1992.

Library of Congress Cataloging-in-Publication Data

Multicultural human services for AIDS treatment and prevention : policy, perspectives, and planning / Julio Morales, Marcia Bok, editors.
     p. cm.
     "Has also been published as Journal of multicultural social work ; volume 2, number 3, 1992"-T.p. verso.
     Includes bibliographical references.
     ISBN 978-1-56024-414-1 (hbk).-ISBN 978-1-56023-038-0 (pbk)
     1. AIDS (Disease-Prevention- Social aspects-United States 2. AIDS (Dis- ease-Treatment-Social aspects-United States. 3. Minorities-Health and hygiene-United States. 4. Minorities-Medical care-United States. 5. Community health service-United States-Cross cultural studies. 6. Social work with minorities-United States. I. Morales, Julio, 1942- .Il. Bok, Marcia. m. Title: Journal of multicultural social work.
     [DNLM: 1. Acquired Immunodeficiency Syndrome-prevention& control. 2. Attitude to Health. 3. Community Health Services-organization & administration-United States. 4. Ethnic Groups-United States. WD 308 M955]
RA644.A25M855 1992
362.1969792'008693-dc20
DNLM/DLC
for Library of Congress   92-48833
                                                  CIP

Multicultural Human Services for AIDS Treatment and Prevention: Policy, Perspectives, and Planning

CONTENTS

ABOUT THE EDITORS

Julio Morales, PhD, is a full professor at the University of Connecticut School of Social Work where he also served as Dean of Students between 1981 and 1984. He has served on the faculty of Brooklyn College and Boston University and created human service agencies or programs in New York, Massachusetts and Connecticut. Dr. Morales has served on the Executive Committee of the Board of Directors of the Urban League of Greater Hartford and serves on the Board of Directors of AIDS Project Hartford. He is currently President of the Board of Latinos(as) Contra SIDA (Latinos Against AIDS). In 1991, Hartford's Hispanic Health Council presented Dr. Morales with their Special Recognition Award for community service; he was named as an American Leadership Fellow, and was included in *Who's Who Among Hispanic Americans*. In 1992, the Connecticut Chapter of the National Association of Social Workers chose Dr. Morales as Social Worker of the Year. Dr. Morales has served on the Board of Editors of four social work journals, published numerous articles and book chapters and is currently working on a second edition of his book *Puerto Rican Poverty and Migration*.

Marcia Bok, PhD, is Professor Emeritus at the University of Connecticut School of Social Work. She has been a social work educator and researcher for over 25 years. Dr. Bok has done extensive research on teenage pregnancy and dropout prevention. She has taught courses in political systems, urban policy, social welfare policy and research in Puerto Rican Studies. Dr. Bok has published in *The Journal of Gerontology, Social Service Review,* and *Affilia: Journal of Women and Social Work.* Her book *Civil Rights and the Social Programs of the 1960's* has recently been released. Dr. Bok is a Board Member of Latinos(as) Contra SIDA. She is a Commissioner on the Permanent Commission on the Status of Women of Hartford and liaison to the Human Relations Commission of the City of Hartford. Drs. Bok and Morales have worked on numerous projects together.

Introduction:
AIDS Within a Cultural Context:
A Perspective

Julio Morales
Marcia Bok

Although it offers the opportunity for intensive closeness and love, and for renewed spirituality and growth, AIDS, as an illness, is often associated with fears and tears, stigma, pity and rejection, loneliness, hatred, anger, alienation and abandonment, dishonor, shame and guilt, frustration, disfigurement, hostility and loss of health, anxiety, depression and discrimination, secrecy and denial, reduced self-esteem, and death. AIDS is an issue which often causes good people to brand others as sinners, instead of focusing on the virus itself. It often intensifies homophobia and forces us to explicitly talk about drugs, sex, and sex workers who are often poor and vulnerable men and women, who rent their bodies for money. When we talk about AIDS, we confront our own values and we expose the inadequacies of medical and other health and human services. The latter is especially important because AIDS, as an illness, has shifted from being equated with instant death to one that people can live with, if motivated and encouraged to seek,

Julio Morales, PhD, is Professor and Marcia Bok, PhD, is Professor Emeritus at the University of Connecticut, School of Social Work, West Hartford, CT 06117.
This introduction contains material from "Puerto Ricans and AIDS: Common Grounds and Concerns," a presentation made by Dr. Julio Morales at Think Thank II–AIDS in Puerto Rico and the Puerto Rican Populations on the Mainland: Care and Treatment of Persons with AIDS–Wednesday, August 22, 1990, San Juan, Puerto Rico.

The editors would like to acknowledge the secretarial support of Elisa Taylor.

obtain and maintain care. At one time, people with AIDS needed care and support for one year or so. Now, they need support and care for many years, making it much harder to maintain secrecy and raising new issues around confidentiality. The growing numbers of people with AIDS, and their increased life expectancy, make obtaining, training, and preventing burn-out among volunteers and paid staff critical. Consciously addressing issues of caring for the care-givers is essential.

The challenges around AIDS are immense and obviously have social, political and economic consequences. As with most chronic illnesses and disabling conditions, if one is not already poor before becoming a person with AIDS, one will become poor in a few years unless one is part of the privileged and wealthy elite. This may be the height of cruelty. People who are fighting for their lives often must give up almost all that they own to get medical care. If they are working, their salaries often go for medicine, transportation and housing at the expense of clothing and food. Social and psychological losses compound physical ones. Losses are painful for psychologically, spiritually, and emotionally healthy persons. Imagine how devastating they can be for a person facing life and death issues as well as the stigma of AIDS. The drug addicted person with AIDS has often already been alienated from family and friends. They are likely to be feeling well one day and on a death bed the next day, and yet, there are insufficient drug prevention and rehabilitation services and too many waiting lists for detoxification and residential programs. Furthermore, many of the drug programs that do exist are usually at risk of budget cuts and are not prepared to treat the addict who uses heroine and cocaine or crack. In addition, few programs are prepared to deal with women and their infected and addicted babies. Too often, the drug addict with AIDS must go back home, a place where he or she may have been rejected previously.

People who have been poor have long been limited to the overburdened and poorly staffed clinics and hospital emergency rooms which have never been able to keep up with their patient loads and demands. The poorest, the most vulnerable and most isolated of the people with AIDS often fall between gaps in services and move from the hospitals to the streets and the ranks of the homeless.

Furthermore, persons who are HIV positive but asymptomatic usually do not qualify for reimbursable services and when they do, they are forced to address issues of confidentiality.

These and other psychosocial issues continue to make AIDS an important substantive area of study for health professionals, including social workers. These common grounds and concerns apply to most people with AIDS regardless of gender or mode of transmission. They may, however, affect different groups of people differently.

The disease has hit Puerto Ricans, Mexican Americans, and other Latinos, African Americans and other racial and ethnic minorities especially hard. Furthermore, it is essential to look at AIDS within a cultural context, to share and encourage research that addresses AIDS and minority populations, and to assess prevention, education and behavioral change strategies from culturally specific and relevant perspectives. This collection does that.

The volume contains articles on African Americans, Native American Indians, Native Hawaiians and Puerto Ricans, all groups who became involuntary citizens of the United States. African Americans were forced to come to the U.S. as slaves, sold in the market place as goods, and unlike European immigrants, faced thousands of laws and barriers that kept them apart and legally blocked opportunities for equality. A history of genocide and hostile and violent takeovers of land and resources is an important perspective to validate and inform social work practice with Native Americans. Puerto Rico and Hawaii were taken by the U.S. in 1898. Puerto Ricans and Hawaiians also share a common history of colonization and forced citizenship. The history and colonial exploitation of Puerto Ricans and Native Hawaiians is essential to understand as it continues to affect both groups.

El Paso and other American Cities were part of Mexico, as was approximately one third of American soil, until the mid-nineteenth century. Many persons of Mexican heritage, like Native Hawaiians, Puerto Ricans, African Americans and Native American Indians, also became involuntary citizens of America. This reality, the geographic sharing of our borders, and the racial mixture of Mexicans distinguish Mexican Americans in the United States from Americans whose ancestors immigrated from Europe. By comparison to

Americans of European heritage, Mexican Americans are disproportionately poor. Indeed, Native Americans, Puerto Ricans, African Americans, Native Hawaiians, and Mexican Americans are
America's poorest ethnic groups. The uniqueness of these people
of color, within American history, is a powerful explanation of the
poverty which they have faced and continue experiencing, in the
U.S. Unfortunately, poverty has become the best predictor of
AIDS. Notice the rapid increase of the epidemic in Africa, Latin
America and developing countries.

Racism, unrelieved poverty, and the social ills that are part of
the definition of poverty, lead to what has been described as the
"full plate syndrome," with AIDS being just one more problem on
that plate. It may not even be the main problem if it competes with
seeking shelter or feeding one's children. Poverty and violence
contribute to the use of drugs as a means of escaping the pain,
leading to greater HIV infection. Poverty, also by definition, means
high levels of stress, malnutrition, housing overcrowding, homelessness, unemployment, dependence, poor education, poor access
to prevention information, etc., all of which are AIDS related.

Color, disproportionate poverty, racism, and a history of con-
quest and forced citizenship make these groups very different from
the European peasants whose children form the U.S. majority
today.

Also different is the cultural context of AIDS. For example,
Hispanics may have a greater judgmental attitude regarding homo-
sexuality than other groups. A component of homophobia is the
failure to address prevention and care as related to Hispanic men
who have sex with other men and who do not identify themselves
as gay or bisexual. This secrecy, coupled with sexism, make Hispanic women less likely to assert themselves or insist on safer sex,
thus being placed at greater risk. Other cultural aspects, like a
fatalistic approach to life, may further impact Hispanics and AIDS.
Emphasis on respect, honor, dignity, hospitality, family, personal-
ismo, confianza, etc., can also play a significant role on how Hispanic families deal with people with AIDS.

Several articles in this edition deal with knowledge, attitudes,
and behavior regarding AIDS among different racial and ethnic
groups. *Vital and Health Statistics* from the U.S. Department of

Health and Human Services, Center for Disease Control, National Center for Health Statistics (October, 1991) provide the following information for blacks and three Hispanic subgroups (Puerto Ricans in the U.S., people of Mexican origin in the U.S., and other Hispanics).

More black, Hispanic and white women than men believe there is no chance of their getting AIDS. Overall, 73 percent of Hispanic adults and 71 percent of black adults feel there is no chance of their becoming infected with HIV. Only 2 percent of Hispanics and whites and 3 percent of blacks reported being in any of the behavior categories associated with a high risk of AIDS. These figures are relatively unchanged from 1988, suggesting that denial of at-risk behaviors continues to be prevalent among all groups.

Among blacks and Hispanics (and the U.S. population as a whole) the greatest levels of knowledge about AIDS occur among the young and well-educated. During 1990, 88 percent of black and Hispanic adults reported having received information about AIDS, with television being the most frequently cited source (77 percent). Information derived from reading material is associated with formal educational levels. Unfortunately, educational levels in the United States (and elsewhere) are not evenly distributed among ethnic, racial or class lines.

Self-assessed knowledge about AIDS also varies with education. The proportion of black and Hispanic adults who correctly identified the major modes of AIDS transmission was relatively high for all socioeconomic groups. However, generally high levels of misperception about the likelihood of transmission through casual contact continues. Changes in knowledge from 1988 to 1990 were particularly noted in the following areas: an increase in those who were aware of drugs available which could extend the life of the HIV infected person and greater awareness that individuals could have the AIDS virus but not the AIDS disease.

While levels of formal education provide explanations for AIDS knowledge, it is important to consider other variables when interpreting knowledge related statistics. For example, all national studies demonstrate that Puerto Ricans have less formal education than most other Latino groups and that as a group Puerto Ricans also lag behind blacks and whites in educational attainment. Nevertheless, CDC data report that 32 percent of Puerto Rican adults rated condoms as "very effective" in preventing AIDS transmission compared with only 22 percent of Mexicans or other Hispanics, 28 percent of blacks, and 27 percent of whites. This, too, was attributed to education.

Furthermore, while 70 percent of non-Hispanic white and black parents with children between the age of 10 and 17 years reported that they ever discussed AIDS with their children, this was true of 50 percent of Mexican-origin parents, 74 percent of Puerto Rican parents, and 64 percent of other Hispanics. Parents discussing AIDS with their children is strongly associated with parental education and gender, with women more likely to discuss AIDS with their children than men.

Given that in education, and in most socio-economic indicators, Puerto Ricans fare worst than almost every other ethnic and racial group in the United States, CDC research leads to questions of data interpretation. Could it be that CDC data are capturing exposure to AIDS information in cities like New York, Boston, and Hartford where Puerto Ricans are concentrated and where there is an extremely high incidence of AIDS? CDC data report that almost one-third (30 percent) of Puerto Ricans had ever known someone with AIDS compared with 19 percent of other Hispanics, 10 percent of persons of Mexican origin, and 18 percent of blacks. In the U.S., Puerto Ricans are almost exclusively dwellers of inner cities of the Northeast. Nationwide their numbers (2.7 million) are small by comparison to blacks (31.4 million), or persons of Mexican origin (13.1 million). At times, population concentrations and regional comparisons offer information which may be more reliable than nationwide data.

Evidence suggests that Puerto Ricans are among the hardest hit group of people in the United States and its territories. For example, in terms of new AIDS cases reported per 100,000 people, for the 12 months ending March of 1990, San Juan was second only to San Francisco, and Puerto Rico led all the states in the mainland. In the June, 1990 edition of the *Journal of Acquired Immune Deficiency Syndrome*, Dr. Barbara Menendez reports that the male AIDS mortality rate in New York City is highest among Puerto Rican migrants, even when compared to other Latinos, African-

Americans or whites. Puerto Ricans in the United States have an AIDS incidence 7 times higher than whites. AIDS has very disproportionately touched the lives of Puerto Rican families and neighborhoods.

Could it be that since AIDS has hit Puerto Ricans so hard, Puerto Rican families are forced to address AIDS from a personal perspective and that it is that explanation, and not formal levels of education, that explain some CDC statistics? Clearly, research is important. Equally important are their implications, interpretations and additional questions which are generated.

THE ARTICLES

"Cultural Dissonance and AIDS in the Puerto Rican Community," the article by Marcia Bok and Julio Morales, addresses cultural issues related to AIDS and Puerto Ricans in Hartford, Connecticut. Some Puerto Rican PWAs feel that cultural characteristics, and the stigma of AIDS, have had the effect of isolating them from their families. However, others feel that those same cultural patterns are the reasons for family support and care. Bok and Morales explore cultural dissonance as they interview social workers, other health professionals and various segments of Hartford's Puerto Rican community.

In "AIDS: Assessing African American Knowledge and Attitudes for Community Education Programs," Debra Moehle McCallum, Joan E. Esser-Stuart, Alyce Vyann Howell and David L. Klemmack, compare and contrast two studies dealing with changes in knowledge, attitudes and behavior over a two year period. One study was done in 1988 and the other in 1990. The data were collected primarily from African Americans throughout Alabama. A random telephone survey and a second survey targeting populations in predominantly black colleges, community health centers, vocational schools, community action agencies and state prisons are discussed. Knowledge, attitudes and behavior changed over the two years and some segments of the population appeared to have more knowledge and more tolerance than others. The authors discuss education and prevention programs and a growing tolerance for

AIDS and homosexuals. They address the importance of using surveys to help develop appropriate AIDS education and prevention programs and to provide knowledge for the researcher while raising awareness and a desire to learn for the persons being interviewed.

In "AIDS in the Native Hawaiian Community," Noreen Mokuau and Alyson Kau address knowledge, attitudes, lifestyle practices and recommendation for services from the perspective of Native Hawaiians. The isolation of the Native Hawaiian is discussed as is the general health and economic status of Native Hawaiians. Viewed in the context of overall poverty and poor health, the authors express concern about the increasing HIV infection risks and identify recommendation that may lead to the development of culturally responsive AIDS programs targeting Native Hawaiians.

The fourth group of involuntary citizens written about in this special issue are Native American Indians. Reportedly, the predominant drug abused in Native American Indian culture is alcohol and the major form of HIV transmission among the Native American population in rural Maine is unprotected sex. Elizabeth DePoy and Claire Bolduc, the authors of "AIDS Prevention in a Rural Native American Population: An Empirical Approach to Program Development," illuminate the importance of social work research for intervention strategies. The authors stress that accurate knowledge and the best intentions are not enough in addressing behavioral change. Ultimately, it is behavioral change that will stop the spread of AIDS. Intervention strategies must be relevant to the beliefs, norms, values and behaviors of the population which is to benefit from the intervention. Based on their research findings DePoy and Bolduc propose a prevention program and discuss the implications for multicultural social work perspectives as related to preventing AIDS.

Prostitution, AIDS and an international border community are the topic of "A Survey of AIDS Knowledge and Attitudes Among Prostitutes in an International Border Community," by Felipe Peralta, Patricia A. Sandau-Beckler and Rosario H. Torres. Prostitutes engage in high risk behavior for AIDS transmission and prostitutes, in this study, generally did not utilize risk reduction behavior while engaging in sex for money. Thus, they are highly vulnerable for receiving HIV and for transmitting the virus. This paper discusses the international problem of the spread of AIDS through prostitution. Knowledge, attitudes and behavior changes among prostitutes, the implication for their clients, themselves, and their children are the themes of this work. The women in the study were prostitutes because they are poor; they view prostitution as a job. Social workers generally do not reach out to this highly alienated group and our own values regarding prostitution may enhance the neglect.

Women who are infected through prostitution, those infected by their husbands or partners, and others who are infected through intravenous drug use may also have children. HIV infected mothers, especially in the later stages of the infection, must be helped in planning for their own children who survive them. "Perinatal AIDS: Permanency Planning for the African American Community," by Susan Taylor-Brown, Chris Wilczynski, Ellen Moore, and Flossie Cohen, highlights the issues which social workers must consider when planning for children who survive their infected parents. The authors discuss culturally appropriate services for empowering parents, particularly African American mothers, as they struggle with the pain and anguish of leaving their children orphaned. Enlisting family members in the care of surviving children and welfare policies affecting kinship foster care and adoption are explored. Strategies for community outreach to assure that African American children remain in the African American community are presented and advocacy and training needs are discussed. The authors review models that calculate future projections of orphaned children as a result of maternal HIV infection and present their own projections. Assisting HIV infected mothers to remain connected to their children and to plan for them is a critical issue that has not received sufficient attention by social workers and other human service providers. Some children are infected while some of their siblings are not. The authors conclude that essential research should lead to a more responsive and appropriate care system for these orphaned children and their families.

The article by Victor De La Cancela and Audrey McDowell, "AIDS: Health Care Intervention Models for Communities of Color," argues that AIDS intervention must include multicultural community based organizational involvement. The authors list a series of potentially effective policy initiatives and a number of concrete interventions that appropriately embrace the sociocultural and political realities of specific groups. For example, De La Cancela and McDowell state that women of color may avoid treatment for fear of losing their children, or having their HIV infected children excluded from schools. How can such people be reached? AIDS, in itself, may prevent AIDS services. The authors explore two themes: The special prevention and treatment needs of people of color and the advantages of community health centers for AIDS treatment rather than acute care in general hospitals.

All the manuscripts indicate that there is significant knowledge about AIDS and attitudes related to the illness are more positive in the 1990s than in the mid or late 1980s. Still, not all people have facts and knowledge, and having this information does not necessarily lead to behavior change. The remaining percentage of people who are uninformed or misinformed about AIDS indicate the need for an intensive effort to reach these individuals with linguistically and culturally targeted educational approaches. In order to change behavior, a multicultural perspective is needed. While knowledge has increased and attitudes have become more tolerant, there is still much to be done in preventing AIDS and reducing risk behaviors in minority communities in the U.S.

Additional research in motivating and maintaining behavior change is essential. Differences within groups (as well as between groups) may call for different approaches in prevention, education, and intervention. Religious beliefs, age, gender, sexual orientation, social class, educational levels and rural/urban differences may be as important to consider as differences between racial and ethnic groups. Clearly, rigorous comparisons between groups to determine multicultural similarities and differences which could lead to more effective prevention and treatment strategies would significantly contribute to practice. Stereotypes, prejudices and negative valuation of gays, people of color, drug users and prostitutes must be continuously addressed. Persons with membership in several disenfranchised groups (i.e., Latino, gay, drug users or black prostitutes with AIDS) may face additional isolation and rejection and may require a more complex array of support and intervention strategies.

Among the policy implications of a multicultural approach are: (1) coordination of services between mainstream and community-based organizations specifically designed to reach minority populations; (2) recognizing AIDS as a priority with sufficient resources allocated for such services as drug treatment, to reduce risk and to provide treatment for infected populations; (3) dissemination and transfer of knowledge about effective prevention and treatment strategies for different population groups; (4) specifying, in more operational terms, what is meant by "culturally sensitive interventions" such as involvement of families as partners in prevention and care, use of indigenous workers, and other bilingual and bicultural concerns. Issues of confidentiality, mandatory testing, needle exchange programs, sex education and distribution of condoms in schools continue to be some of the subjects for debate which reflect the political nature of AIDS. Thus, social workers need to understand and influence policies and political processes, as well as engaging in direct practice. The ramifications of AIDS are so multifaceted that only the most inclusive approach to understanding and treating the disease can be effective.

While the guest editors believe that the articles in this volume make an important contribution to understanding AIDS, we also believe that the material reflects a beginning effort to explicate the many intricate issues in multicultural social work with individuals, families and communities affected by HIV/AIDS. The research is often exploratory but it illustrates the status of social work research in this area. Thus, the material presented is considered a foundation which will lead to further research, investigation, and understanding of the complex nature of AIDS.

Cultural Dissonance and AIDS in the Puerto Rican Community

Marcia Bok
Julio Morales

SUMMARY. Puerto Ricans with AIDS constitute a distinct ethnic group and illustrate the need for a multicultural approach to social work practice with individuals with HIV infection and AIDS. This paper deals with the dissonance created when cultural characteristics of nurturance, support, and caring clash with feelings of fear, stigma, and anger and cause conflict in the helping process.

INTRODUCTION

The AIDS epidemic, considered by many as a modern-day plague, has disproportionately affected the Hispanic population and other people of color. Although Hispanics comprise only 8 percent of the population in the United States, they constitute 16 percent of the adult AIDS population; and while African-Americans comprise 11 percent of the population, they account for 27 percent of adult cases of AIDS. Among children with AIDS, 25 percent are Hispanic and 53 percent are African-American (CDC, 1990). Within the Hispanic community, AIDS strikes most heavily among poor, intravenous drug users and their sexual partners and children.

This paper deals with Puerto Ricans, who are the largest Hispanic group in the Northeast, and specifically Puerto Ricans in the Hart-

Marcia Bok, PhD, is Professor Emeritus and Julio Morales, PhD, is Professor, University of Connecticut, School of Social Work, West Hartford, CT 06117.

13

ford area in Connecticut. The findings of the paper are based on exploratory interviews within the Puerto Rican community, as well as observations of services provided and utilized by Puerto Ricans infected and affected by HIV and AIDS. The large number of families with HIV and AIDS within the Puerto Rican community, with many women and children requiring treatment, as well as women as caregivers participating in support groups, contrasts sharply with the requirements for care within the gay, white community. These differences are only one example of the many faceted, multicultural requirements of AIDS that need to be addressed (see Carillo, 1988).

The Puerto Rican family is generally acknowledged as loving, caring, and nurturing (Mizio, 1981; Morales, 1992). These characteristics have endured despite family disruptions caused by poverty, dislocations from rural to urban settings, and migration between the United States and Puerto Rico. But the Puerto Rican also tends to be moralistic and traditional in family values and fatalistic toward conditions and events perceived to be beyond the individual's control. Behaviors such as drug abuse, prostitution and homosexuality are generally maligned within the Puerto Rican community. This negative attribution leads to social denial which makes prevention of at-risk behaviors more difficult (See Fullilove, 1989); and interferes with willingness to provide and seek help when HIV or AIDS is present (See McDonell et al., 1991). Worth and Rodriguez (1987) note that fear and denial may destabilize the usually nurturing extended family support network resulting in isolation and even homelessness for Latinos(as) with AIDS. Therefore, based on prejudice and stigma toward the behaviors associated with HIV and AIDS, on the one hand, yet inclined to be nurturing, on the other, the Puerto Rican individual and family are caught in a response dilemma in regard to the disease. This cultural dissonance–that is, conflict between opposing attitudes, beliefs, and behaviors which are internalized and create individual and interpersonal stress–presents a unique opportunity to understand how personal and cultural inconsistencies are resolved in the helping process. Thus, this paper begins to explore ways that Puerto Ricans perceive HIV and AIDS and efforts by the community to cope with the individual and cultural dissonance created by the disease.

RESEARCH METHODOLOGY

Between 1988 and 1990, the authors gathered data from the Puerto Rican community in the Hartford area about experiences and attitudes toward AIDS. M.S.W. students and faculty from the Puerto Rican Studies Project[1] at the University of Connecticut School of Social Work participated in these exploratory efforts. Almost all the students and faculty who designed the research instruments and conducted the interviews were Puerto Rican and bilingual and bicultural in Spanish and English. Interviews included Puerto Ricans with HIV and AIDS, service providers, community people, and family members impacted by HIV and AIDS. These exploratory interviews brought to light the conflicts within the Puerto Rican community about the meaning and implications of HIV and AIDS and provided direction for the continuation of research in this area. As already suggested, the data reported below provide some insights, but are considered very tentative and raise as many questions as are answered.

The multi-stage research project, in which the students and faculty from the Puerto Rican Studies Project participated, began with interviews with Puerto Ricans with HIV and AIDS in 1988. At that time, the social work community in Connecticut was just beginning to address the needs of individuals with the disease and few social service resources were available. A crisis in the demand for care and issues of confidentiality, together with a general reluctance of clinical social workers to engage in research, made it very difficult to gather data from people with HIV and AIDS (PWAs).

Health care professionals were interviewed in 1989. These findings supplement data derived from PWA and provide an additional perspective on the perception of AIDS within the Puerto Rican community.

In 1990, interviews were conducted in the community with two groups of Puerto Ricans: (1) church-goers interviewed by students at Pentacostal and Roman Catholic church sites following church services; and (2) interviews with Puerto Rican proprietors (and a few employees) in small stores (e.g., bodegas, beauty shops, record stores, clothing stores) along Park Street, a commercial strip concentrated with Puerto Rican merchants. Additional students were enlisted for these efforts. A small number of relatives of PWA were also interviewed in 1990.

In the analysis of the data, rigorous statistical tests are not applied for comparisons between groups because interviews were meant to be exploratory. Continued research in this area should strive for greater rigor, such as random sampling, and should use tests of statistical significance to increase confidence in the meaning of research results.

In the interviews, many different kinds of questions about HIV and AIDS were asked. Although related questions are included, the analysis of data in this paper focuses mainly on questions related to the helping process and attitudes related to helping. This includes: perceived attitudes toward people with AIDs and family members with AIDS; how the role of professionals and family members as helpers is perceived; perceived differences between Puerto Ricans and non-Puerto Ricans in helping family members with AIDS; and differences in support systems within the Puerto Rican community around AIDS and other illnesses.

FINDINGS

People with AIDS (PWA)

Over a period of three years, a total of 35 personal, face-to-face interviews with PWA were completed. Seventy-four percent of respondents were male and 26 percent female; 57 percent were seropositive and 43 percent had AIDS. Forty-eight percent had contracted the virus through intravenous drug use; 26 percent from homosexual contact; and 26 percent from heterosexual activities with infected partners. Seventy-eight percent of the women had contracted the disease from an infected partner.

Interviews with PWA revealed many changes in their lives. This includes changes in marital status, employment, living arrangements, social contacts, and, of course, health status. Respondents reported they had changed nutritional habits, exercised more, cut down on alcohol and drug use, and changed their sexual behavior.

Although in most situations families were supportive, particularly siblings, not all family members or friends were necessarily informed about the individual's health status, particularly if the individual was asymptomatic. For example, very elderly parents living in Puerto Rico might be protected. There was a considerable degree of self-imposed isolation and some individuals were reluctant to reveal their HIV or AIDS status to everyone. Most PWA said they were making efforts not to spread the disease through safer sex, through total abstinence from sexual activity, or by avoidance of contact with family members and friends (which was part of the self-imposed isolation). Many were also avoiding friends and relatives who were associated with drug use. Generally, PWAs were ashamed of having HIV or AIDS. Many stated they feared rejection and reprisal, that they were protecting others and that they were depressed. Furthermore, because modes of transmission of the virus were not well understood, they were often alone unnecessarily. In situations of drug abuse, respondents may have already been estranged from parents and other relatives and actual rejection by some family members, particularly spouse or companeras, did occur. Most often, however, these responses were complex. While some spouses might be totally estranged, others might avoid sexual contact but be helpful and supportive in other ways.

Over 90 percent of PWA did not think the health care they were receiving was different because they were Puerto Rican; and 65 percent believed that people did not react differently toward them because they were Puerto Rican. However, 32 percent thought they were treated worse (i.e., more rejected than non-Puerto Ricans).

With regard to help provided by social workers, many appreciative sentiments were expressed. However, early in the interviewing, social workers were not yet heavily immersed in treatment of PWA; help was mainly provided by other health professionals, such as nurses and doctors and drug counselors. Several respondents indicated that social workers were slow to cut through bureaucratic red-tape which prevented them from receiving needed income or health care in a timely fashion, also indicating newness to the issues of AIDS.

Service Providers

Interviews with 34 health care professionals who were white (27 percent), Puerto Rican (70 percent), and other Hispanic (3 percent) working with Puerto Ricans with HIV and AIDS, were conducted in 1989.

Contrary to the assessment by PWA, 56 percent of health professionals thought the quality of health care for Puerto Ricans and non-Puerto Ricans with AIDS was different. It was felt that services were less available to Puerto Ricans, especially those on welfare. Providers also felt that there were few bilingual and bicultural staff and that discrimination and racism existed. Thirty-two percent were not certain if there were differences in quality of care.

All of the service providers believed there were moral and judgmental attitudes toward AIDS in the society. Sixty-two percent believed this was stronger in the Puerto Rican community; 44 percent believed that Puerto Ricans with AIDS were more stigmatized in their community than non-Puerto Ricans in their communities. However, 32 percent of respondents were uncertain about the answer to this question. A large number of service providers also revealed their own negative attitudes toward PWA. (These findings are reinforced by other researchers, as well. See Wiener and Siegel, 1990 and Miller and Carlton, 1988.)

Fifty-three percent of service providers believed that Puerto Rican families were involved a great deal in the care of family members with AIDS; 41 percent thought families were somewhat involved. Two-thirds of respondents thought Puerto Rican families were different that non-Puerto Ricans in their response to family members with AIDS, with 52 percent believing that Puerto Ricans were more compassionate, more nurturing, more understanding, and more supportive. Twenty-two percent thought Puerto Ricans might turn away from family members with AIDS because they were fearful and less knowledgeable about the disease.

When asked if the traditional Puerto Rican network of extended family support is destabilized (i.e., disrupted) in situations of AIDS, 65 percent of respondents thought this was true, at least initially or due to burnout after a long period of illness and intense care; 24 percent said no; and 11 percent were uncertain or did not know. The comments to this question were most revealing:

> "Initially disrupted while adjusting to the shock of the diagnosis";
>
> "The nuclear family takes on the burden of responsibility and other family members turn away",
>
> "If Cousin Pedro is sick everyone goes into a frenzy; there is a lot of shock, a lot of anguish, a lot of anger, but they support . . . "
>
> "They are willing to help and accept the HIV/AIDS person, but they are afraid of AIDS itself."

Additional comments about "denial and concealment of the true diagnosis," "fear of contagion, lack of knowledge, fear of death," "isolating patient from children," and "because they are afraid sometimes family does not function well. . . ." further illustrate the contradictory impulses that pull Puerto Ricans in different directions simultaneously around AIDS. Most important from a social work perspective was the belief of service providers that Puerto Rican families need outside help and support to deal with the initial shock of the diagnosis, to provide needed information, and to prevent burnout in the long haul ahead.

Community Respondents

Sixty-three interviews with church-goers and 40 with small shop-keepers were completed. Over three-fourths of church-goers indicated they were interested in learning more about AIDS. Shopkeepers generally thought their customers are somewhat interested in learning more about AIDS, but that customers are reluctant to talk about it. Over 50 percent of church-goers believed it would not be difficult to educate the Puerto Rican community about AIDS, but 29 percent thought it would be difficult. Eighty-eight percent of shop-keepers would be willing to distribute literature on AIDS in their stores.

Fifty-nine percent of church-goers and 74 percent of shopkeepers believe that AIDS brings shame to the Puerto Rican family because of the way it is transmitted. Other respondents were uncertain about their response to this question. Both groups of respondents believe that a family's initial reaction to learning about AIDS in the family would be disbelief and shock, anger, pity, fear, sadness and compassion, and acceptance and willingness to help, if possible. Eighty percent of shop-keepers mentioned fear and 65 percent identified pity (in an open-ended question).

Forty-eight percent of shop-keepers and 35 percent of churchgoers did not believe that Puerto Ricans would react differently than non-Puerto Ricans to a family member with AIDS. Only 28 percent of shop-keepers thought the help provided to family members with AIDS would be different in the Puerto Rican family. "Family is family." This contrasts with two-thirds of service providers who thought Puerto Ricans would react differently, and this would be, mainly, in the direction of greater compassion. But church-goers were particularly uncertain about the answer to this question. Thirty-seven percent of church-goers thought the support system for Puerto Ricans would be different for AIDS and other illnesses, but many (40 percent) were uncertain about their response. Forty-five percent of shop-keepers believed support would be different for AIDS and other illnesses.

Family Reactions

Based on a very small number of interviews (N = 5) with Puerto Ricans in Hartford with PWA in the family, the following findings are suggested. While a great deal of change occurs in all areas of life as a result of AIDS, one major change occurs in living arrangements. Husbands and wives and companeros (as) are separated; patients move in with parents or other family members; patients live alone during some part of their long, chronic illness.

Family members recall reactions of denial, anger, sadness, guilt, confusion and pain, acceptance, and intense fear, especially in relation to sexual contact with PWA. Most respondents thought AIDS brought families together, but respondents indicated that not all family members knew about the illness. Almost all respondents believed that their reaction to AIDS would be the same as with other illnesses: "We would be there for him" (although community respondents thought it might be different). Complex reactions are suggested by a companera who left her companero because he had AIDS; she refused sexual contact, but visited frequently and provided as much help and support as possible. A mother whose daughter had AIDS visited the daughter constantly in the hospital. When she brought food, however, she used "sterilized," separate utensils. She also refused to take her daughter home from the hospital because she was caring for her grandchildren and feared contagion.

Summary of Findings

PWA indicate a great deal of self-imposed isolation based on shame, depression, fear of rejection, and fear of spreading the disease. Some rejection is real, especially from spouse and companero(a), but support is also forthcoming, particularly from siblings and other family members. In many situations, especially where the individual is seropositive but not ill with AIDS, the individuals tend not to reveal their health status to many people who might be helpful or rejecting.

Service providers universally believe that society is moralistic and judgmental regarding AIDS and Puerto Ricans may be even more moralistic. Over 50 percent believe that Puerto Ricans are greatly involved in the health care of family members with AIDS; and 52 percent believe Puerto Ricans are more compassionate, nurturing, understanding, and supportive of family members with AIDS than non-Puerto Ricans. Almost two-thirds believe the Puerto Rican family is destabilized–disrupted–at least initially by AIDS.

Community respondents agree that AIDS brings shame to families. But they also believe Puerto Ricans are not different from other people in their reaction to family members with AIDS and the help they provide–"Family is family"–(note different perception by service providers). However, community respondents thought the family support system within the Puerto Rican community might be different for AIDS compared with other illnesses.

AIDS forces many changes on families; and change in living arrangements is one frequent occurrence. Families obviously have many different and intense reactions to learning about a family member with AIDS, but fear is prevalent. Families are likely to pull together around AIDS and "be there" for the individual who is ill. But reactions are complex and often ambivalent.

One family member was offended because the interviewer asked how AIDS was contracted by his brother. "Why do you ask people how they got AIDS? You wouldn't ask people how they got cancer!" Good point! As Sontag (1989) emphasizes, AIDS is so much of a metaphor for other bad conditions in life that we lose sight of the fact that AIDS is an illness that can be prevented, treated, and eventually cured and eliminated, like any other illness. That agenda is often overlooked because of the many layers of unreality attached to the disease.

DISCUSSION

A May 17, 1989 column in the *Hartford Courant* contained the following dire message: "Candidly, I don't know that I've seen a lot of sympathy even for the gays" . . . "but in the hierarchy of things, the intravenous drug user is at the bottom of the list. I don't know how that will change, but there are major racial and class attitudes that have to be overcome to deal with this problem" . . . "Sometimes the racial and class issues at work in this are overwhelming. There are serious things here, and I'm not sure there's the political will to redress them."

That was in 1989. We think we have made progress since then, with more education, more understanding, more tolerance and more acceptance of people with AIDS. But AIDS will certainly not heal the wounds of ethnocentricity, racism, homophobia, and classism in the society and, thus, there continues to be a crucial need for a multicultural perspective to deal with the AIDS crisis.

There is a general lack of research on the multicultural, psychosocial aspects of AIDS. This paper specifically tries to highlight some of the issues that complicate the perception, attitudes, and treatment of AIDS in the Puerto Rican community. We have seen how fear, pity, anger, and compassion are some of the complex and contradictory emotions that AIDS engenders. We have tried to illustrate, in a limited way, how the Puerto Rican community is coping with these dilemmas. Although the authors believe that the findings of the research and the questions raised in this paper are significant, many questions remain.

The data suggest a great deal of uncertainty in responses from almost all of the populations interviewed. Lack of direct experience with AIDS can account for some of this uncertainty. It would be particularly difficult for respondents to compare reactions of Puerto Ricans and non-Puerto Ricans when there is limited contact across racial and ethnic groups. In Hartford and elsewhere, blacks, Puerto Ricans, and whites live in separate communities and adults in different groups have little interaction with each other. As a result, each may not have information about the other groups. Health professionals may have more multicultural contact, but even health care professionals in 1989 may not have had much experience with different cultural groups with AIDS. The research does not compare attitudes, perceptions, and behaviors of Puerto Ricans and non-Puerto Ricans directly. Thus, the cultural dissonance observed in Puerto Ricans may be present in other groups as well; and similarities, as well as differences, between groups need to be the subject of research.

Obviously no generalizations can be reached from any of the populations interviewed. The church-goers and shop-keepers interviewed may not be representative of their respective communities or the total Puerto Rican community with its differences in demographic characteristics. At least two different groups of churchgoers–Pentecostal and Roman Catholic–were interviewed. Even among PWA, the gay population and intravenous drug-users may have very different experiences with the helping process. In the rapidly changing situation of AIDS, attitudes might be very different in 1992 than two or three years ago.

Further theory in this area is also needed. The theoretical work of McDonell et al. (1991) which attempts to develop a predictive paradigm for "willingness to help" suggests that the concept of cultural dissonance could also be applied to measure helping behavior. Thus, adding such factors as anger, fear and denial, for example, along with nurturance and compassion, would provide additional information to predict "willingness to help." This kind of information would be useful to assess and compare "willingness to help'' across multicultural lines, with different illnesses, and with different socioeconomic groups.

The findings of the research also suggest some of the ways that social workers can be helpful to the Puerto Rican community around the issues of cultural dissonance. First, social workers need to recognize and understand the dilemma. Second, they must be able to verbalize and articulate the dilemma for the individuals and families who are dealing with the dissonance. Third, they must provide knowledge that will reduce some of the fear and anger that is causing the dissonance, because fear and anger are some of the barriers to acceptance and love. And finally, they must allow clients and patients to express their ambivalence, and negative, as well as positive feelings. An acknowledgement and reduction in dissonance will relieve a great deal of stress and tension within individuals and among family members trying to cope with AIDS. For example, family members who are not able to be truthful with each other experience additional stress and estrangement. Interpersonal tensions certainly exacerbate physical illness and openness between family members can provide some relief.

Other social work roles include helping HIV and PWA to reveal their health status to friends and relatives so that needed support can be forthcoming. Where patients are estranged from their families because of homosexuality or drug use, social workers can help to reconnect family members where this is desired and feasible. Social workers can provide support to individuals and families through individual counseling and peer support groups to strengthen existing resources and prevent burn-out as the illness lingers and worsens. Concrete tasks, case management and advocacy roles, and public policy responsibilities are also needed. Clearly, social workers can provide the encouragement that is needed to sustain hope and optimism for the future.

In the authors' experiences, in working with Puerto Ricans with AIDS, the needs of Puerto Rican women and children and whole families are particularly acute. This is often overlooked in AIDS research and literature. Some organizations, such as Latinos(as) Contra SIDA, in Hartford, Connecticut, deal with AIDS as a family issue. Nationally, over 15,000 cases of AIDS in women have been reported, more than 10 percent of the total. It is estimated that more than 100,000 women are infected with the virus. Women are the fastest growing category of people with AIDS in the United States (Stuntzner-Gibson, 1991). Yet women are often blamed for infecting their children or their sexual partners and have not received enough attention on their own behalf.

Although African-American and Hispanic women constitute 19 percent of all U.S. women, they represent 73 percent of all women diagnosed with AIDS (52 percent African-American and 21 percent Latina). Among adolescent AIDS cases, 38 percent are female.

It is estimated that in New York City, by 1993, there will be 20,000 children who have lost their mothers to AIDS. Puerto Ricans will be overrepresented in this group. Many of these women are single parents. Given current projections, by the year 2000, the number of AIDS orphans will exceed 100,000. In moving research, prevention, treatment, and experimental drug trials onto a higher level, the dilemmas for women and the decisions they need to make should be addressed; and child welfare and family issues must receive utmost attention. A multicultural approach to AIDS is particularly needed to address these concerns.

NOTE

1. The Puerto Rican Studies Project was initially funded by NIMH to recruit, retain, and graduate Puerto Rican and other Latino students with M.S.W. degrees; train social service providers to provide better services to Puerto Ricans; develop curriculum and courses on Puerto Rican client systems; and encourage research and disseminate findings on policy and practice that impact the Puerto Rican community. Much of the original project has been institutionalized into the ongoing M.S.W. program.

REFERENCES

Emilio Carrillo, AIDS and the Latino Community, *Centro,* Centro De Estudios Puertorriguenos, Hunter College, City University of New York, New York, New York, 1988, 2, 4, 7-14.
Centers for Disease Control, March, 1990, U.S. AIDS Cases Reported through February, 1990. *HIV/AIDS Surveillance Report,* 11-18.

Mindy Fullilove, Social Denial: A Barrier to Halting AIDS, *Multicultural Inquiry and Research on AIDS (MIRA)*, Spring, 1989, *3*, 2, 5-6.

James McDonell, Neil Abell, and Jane Miller, Family Members' Willingness to Care for People with AIDS: A Psychosocial Assessment Model, *Social Work*, January, 1991, *36*, 1, 43-53.

Jaclyn Miller and Thomas Carlton, Children and AIDS: A Need to Rethink Child Welfare Practice, *Social Work*, Nov./Dec., 1988, *33*, 6, 553-555.

Emelicia Mizio, Puerto Rican Culture, in E. Mizio and A. Delancy, eds., *Training for Service Delivery to Minority Clients*. New York: Family Service Association of America, 1981.

Julio Morales, Community Social Work in Puerto Rican Communities in the United States; One Organizer's Perspective. in F. Rivera and J. Ehrlich, eds., *Community Organization in a Diverse Society*. Boston: Allyn and Bacon, 1992.

Susan Sontag, *AIDS and its Metaphors*, New York: Farrar, Straus and Giroux, 1989.

Denise Stuntzner-Gibson, Women and HIV Disease: An Emerging Social Crisis, *Social Work*, January, 1991, *36*, 1, 22-28.

Lori Wiener, Women and Human Immunodeficiency Virus: A Historical and Personal Psychosocial Perspective, *Social Work*, September, 1991, *36*, 5, 375-378.

Lori Wiener and Karolynn Siegel, Social Workers' Comfort in Providing Services to AIDS Patients, *Social Work*, January, 1990, *35*, 1, 16-25.

Dooley Worth and Ruth Rodriguez, Latina Women and AIDS, *Radical America*, 1987, *20*, 6, 63-67.

AIDS:
Assessing African-American Knowledge and Attitudes for Community Education Programs

Debra Moehle McCallum
Joan E. Esser-Stuart
Alyce Vyann Howell
David L. Klemmack

SUMMARY. A questionnaire assessing AIDS-related knowledge, attitudes and behaviors was distributed in written form and administered by telephone interviews in 1988 and again in 1990. Data were collected from members of minorities throughout Alabama. The telephone survey was based on a random sample, while the written form was distributed at targeted locations including community health centers, community action agencies, state prisons, vocational schools, and predominantly black colleges. Ninety-four percent of respondents in the telephone survey were African-American, while 84% in the written sample indicated they were African-American. Over the entire sample, knowledge of AIDS transmission was relatively accurate and increased from 1988 to 1990. Knowledge was higher in the written sample than the telephone sample at both

Debra Moehle McCallum, PhD, and Joan E. Esser-Stuart, MSSW, are affiliated with the Institute for Social Science Research at the University of Alabama. Alyce Vyann Howell, BS, is with the Cooperative Health Manpower Education Program at Tuskegee Area Health Education Center, Inc. David L. Klemmack, PhD, is affiliated with the Department of Sociology at the University of Alabama.

The authors thank Liborius Agwara, Kathi Kline, Tom Stem, and Arthur Turner for their assistance with data analysis.

Requests for reprints should be sent to Debra Moehle McCallum, Institute for Social Science Research, P.O. Box 870216, University of Alabama, Tuscaloosa, AL 35487-0216.

27

times. The youngest and oldest age groups were least knowledgeable. In addition to knowledge, other variables including concern about contracting AIDS, behavior change, interest in learning about AIDS, and issues related to stigmatization were investigated. Implications for educational and prevention programs are discussed.

Numerous surveys have been conducted to measure public opinion, knowledge, and behaviors with regard to AIDS. Singer, Rogers, and Corcoran (1987) reviewed twenty-two such surveys conducted between 1983 and 1986. A number of polling organizations, such as Gallup and Roper, have continued to include AIDS questions routinely on national polls. General trends have shown an increase in awareness and knowledge of transmission of AIDS, until by 1988, 92% of respondents knew that AIDS could be transmitted through heterosexual contact, and nearly 100% had accurate knowledge regarding transmission via homosexual contact and sharing of drug needles (Singer, Rogers & Glassman, 1991). On the other hand, misinformation regarding transmission via casual contact is still common (Keppel, Vogt, Brozicevic, & Kutzko, 1989), and very low percentages of individuals indicate any specific behavior changes resulting from their knowledge or fear of AIDS (Singer et al., 1991).

While Singer et al. (1991) reported no overall change in personal worry about AIDS from 1987 to 1988, and a small decrease in worry for those in the age range of 18 to 44 years, it also was apparent that non-whites reported a much higher level of personal concern than whites, and there was a substantial increase in concern over time among non-white respondents. This greater level of concern reflects the reality of the situation, as AIDS is disproportionately high in minority populations. In Alabama, where the current study was conducted, 44% of the reported AIDS cases through June 1991 were African-Americans, although African-Americans comprise just 26% of the state's total population. In 1991, over 50% of the newly reported AIDS cases were African-Americans. In order to combat AIDS in minority groups, it is essential to assess knowledge, attitudes, and behaviors within the community and design programs that will respond specifically to the needs and concerns of these groups. In spite of the potential barriers to obtaining support for such programs in minority communities (Dalton, 1989), a number of such programs are operating effectively throughout the country. The Minorities Prevention of AIDS through Choices and Training (MPACT) Program in Alabama is one such program. MPACT is designed to facilitate change within the lives of minority individuals by using a variety of culturally sensitive educational innovations.

The MPACT Program addresses the minority population via four Area Centers located in different geographical areas throughout the state. Each Area Center is responsible for implementing plans to deliver AIDS and risk-reduction health education to minorities within its geographical target area. One of the major goals for the program is to educate individuals and provide them with knowledge and skills so that they can make positive choices for their lives. This is done partly by identifying leaders within communities and training them to be the bearers of information, rather than relying solely on professional intervention. This indigenous leader approach is similar to that used successfully in other community intervention programs.

In achieving its goals, MPACT has developed an array of education training modules, pamphlets, audio-visual materials, and "training-the-trainer" modules, all of which are minority focused, with specific attention to cultural and language characteristics of the African-American population in Alabama. Numerous professional training sessions and community AIDS education sessions have been conducted since the program began in 1988. When initiating a community AIDS education program, an MPACT Area Coordinator works with a contact person from that community to develop a program tailored specifically for the target audience. Together they design a program which takes into account the reading level, knowledge, language use, specific problems, presence and type of AIDS cases, home settings, sexual activity, and other lifestyle considerations of the participants. The program designed for a church youth group would be different from one designed for a residential drug abuse program, and both would be different from one designed for a group of elderly housing project residents. Similarly, the approach or focus may be different in differing areas of the state, reflecting the diversity of problems in these areas. For example, IV drug use is a major AIDS-related problem in the southern area, teenage pregnancy is a greater problem in the northern area, and an alarming outbreak of syphilis combined with HIV is occurring in the central part of the state. The Area Coordinators are educators, well-established within their communities, and they have received additional training in African-American cultural sensitivity. In the first three years of the program, 24,000 individuals have participated in 350 community education programs, and over 4,000 professionals (health care workers, teachers, social workers, ministers, etc.) have participated in 117 training workshops.

In addition to the training and education sessions, MPACT has worked to develop a statewide mass media campaign on AIDS targeted for special minority populations. This campaign includes print and broadcast media, as well as innovative media productions for youth, such as AIDS Awareness poster contests and AIDS Awareness rap contests. In all of its endeavors, MPACT seeks to assist individuals in making a pact with themselves towards reducing their risk of HIV infection.[1]

The surveys reported in this article were designed by MPACT to assist in determining specific areas of need to be targeted for AIDS education programming. The surveys, intended to investigate the AIDS-related information, attitudes and behaviors among the African-American population in Alabama, were conducted twice–in 1988, before the MPACT program became active, and again two years later in 1990. Because of the lack of appropriate comparisons and controls for extraneous variables, the results cannot provide a direct evaluation or assessment of the MPACT program, nor were they intended to do so. Instead, they were intended as a guide for program development. The results do show, however, some interesting shifts over time in several of the issues of concern to MPACT, as well as areas where little change occurred. These results will be used in the development of future MPACT programs.

METHOD

In the summer of 1988 and again in the summer of 1990, MPACT undertook to survey the non-white population in Alabama with regard to AIDS-related knowledge, attitudes and behavior. The two methods of data collection included a written survey and a telephone survey.

Subjects

Written questionnaires were distributed by the MPACT Program to a variety of sites serving minorities throughout the state. These sites included community health centers, county health departments, community action agencies, state prisons, vocational schools, and colleges with predominantly African-American student bodies. Approximately 4,000 questionnaires were distributed in 1988 and 4,900 were distributed to these sites in 1990. Questionnaires were self-administered and returned anonymously to CHEP/TAHEC or to the area networking agency by those volunteering to participate.

Simultaneously the same set of questions was used to conduct two random-sample telephone surveys during the summers of 1988 and 1990. Random-digit-dialing was used to select household telephone numbers, and within each household an adult respondent was randomly selected. All respondents were asked to identify their race on the sixth item in the survey. Respondents identifying themselves within any group other than White (i.e., Black, Hispanic, Native American, Asian, or Other) were considered minorities and were asked all of the questions that appeared on the written survey. Results from these non-white respondents are reported here. (Interviews with White respondents were terminated shortly after the race identification question.)

In 1988, 1,497 written surveys were returned, and in 1990, 1,465 surveys were returned. The 1988 telephone sample was 501, and the 1990 sample size was 514. Therefore, the total number of participants in the survey was 3,977. The telephone surveys represent random samples among minorities who could be reached by telephone; however, lower income households often are underrepresented in telephone samples (Thornberry & Massey, 1988). Although the written survey samples were focused on specific groups, were not random, and contain no controls for duplicate respondents or for estimating response rates, the demographic information confirms that the written surveys did reach a somewhat different population than the telephone surveys, thus providing valuable and distinctive information.

Questionnaire

The survey consisted of items related to knowledge, attitudes and behaviors regarding AIDS, as well as some demographic information. Items were developed by members of the Alabama AIM program (former name of MPACT) after reviewing a number of instruments used in other AIDS-related surveys (e.g., National Health Interview Survey). Basic questions were selected from this collection of instruments, then modified and structured so as to have a common format and to be understood by a broad segment of the minority population. All items (except demographic variables) were presented with a three-choice format: *Yes, No,* and *Don't know.*

RESULTS

Demographic Information

As mentioned previously, the written and telephone samples do reflect some important differences in demographic variables. In the written sample, 53% were single, 48% reported incomes below $10,000, and 32% were under the age of 22. Eighty-four percent of the written sample indicated they are Black, 2% Hispanic, 5% Native American, .4% Asian, 5% Other, and 4% gave no answer. For the telephone sample, 29% were single, 18% had incomes below $10,000, and 9% were younger than 22 years. (Only individuals 18 years or older were eligible for the telephone survey.) In addition, 94% of the telephone sample indicated they are Black, with less than 2% in any other category. Thirty-four percent of the written sample were male, with 31% males in the telephone sample. Thus the written survey reached a younger, less affluent group, who were more likely to be single. In both samples women were overrepresented. Although the written sample appeared to have somewhat larger representations of minority groups other than

African-Americans, there may have been some confusion regarding the "Native American" designation, some Whites are included in the "Other" category (although Whites were excluded from the telephone survey), and no group is large enough to analyze separately.

Knowledge of AIDS Transmission

Eight items on the questionnaire involved specific knowledge concerning risk-taking behaviors and the transmission of the AIDS virus. Overall the level of knowledge concerning the transmission of AIDS was high in both years and across both formats, and was comparable to that found in national surveys (Singer et al., 1991). More than 90% of the respondents in each sample correctly answered six items concerning the transmission of AIDS through sexual contact and drug needles. Between 85% and 90% in each sample knew that using condoms and spermicides could help prevent the spread of AIDS, but less than 50% in each sample knew that the use of a diaphragm would not prevent the spread of AIDS. This pattern suggests that many respondents may inappropriately equate pregnancy prevention techniques with AIDS prevention techniques.

Respondents were divided into two categories–those who answered all eight knowledge items correctly and those who answered at least one item incorrectly. Results based on this composite measure of knowledge suggest that the level of knowledge about AIDS increased from 1988 to 1990 both in the written samples and the random telephone samples (see Table 1). The results also indicate that those in the written samples had more knowledge than those in the random samples at both survey times.[2]

Because the behavior of various age categories places them at differing levels of risk for contracting AIDS, it is useful to examine the differences in knowledge among these categories. Like national samples (Singer et al., 1991), the relationship between age and knowledge is curvilinear, with statistically significant effects at the $p \leq .05$ level for both of the written samples and the 1988 telephone sample. The 1990 telephone sample shows a marginal effect with $p = .08$. The youngest and the oldest respondents in all four

Table 1

Percentage and Frequency of Respondents Answering All Eight Knowledge Items Correctly

	Written				Telephone			
	1988		1990		1988		1990	
	N = 1487		N = 1450		N = 499		N = 499	
	%	N	%	N	%	N	%	N
Total[a]	59.1	879	64.6	937	43.5	217	51.9	259
< 15 years	36.3	29	40.8	20	---		---	
16-18	50.7	142	53.6	103	44.4	8	47.4	9
19-21	53.6	274	65.3	128	48.0	12	54.5	18
22-30	65.7	359	71.1	236	50.0	51	54.9	67
31-40	70.5	288	74.1	209	54.8	63	62.0	67
>40 years	53.3	122	61.5	278	34.5	79	45.8	98

[a] Written vs. telephone, $p < .05$.
1988 vs. 1990, $p < .05$.
Written, 1988 vs. 1990, $p < .05$;
Telephone, 1988 vs. 1990, $p < .05$;
1988, written vs. telephone, $p < .05$;
1990, written vs. telephone, $p < .05$.

samples are the least knowledgeable, but all age groups show at least some increase in knowledge over time.

Additional Results

More respondents indicated they were worried about AIDS in 1988 (39.8%) than in 1990 (34.5%), and there was no difference in the percentage who had changed their behavior because of their concern (55.7% in both years). As expected, there was a high correspondence between those reporting concern about getting AIDS and those reporting behavior changes. However, there was a small (but statistically reliable at $p \leq .05$) increase in this correspondence from 1988, when 77.0% of those who were worried also indicated some behavior change, to 1990 when this number rose to 80.8%.

Three questions assessed respondents' interest in AIDS information. In 1988 and in 1990, approximately 83% indicated willingness to take a blood test for AIDS. There was a drop from 83.2% in 1988 to 77.9% in 1990 for those who would attend a meeting to learn more about AIDS. Approximately 80% of the respondents (82.2% in 1988 and 79.6% in 1990) reported that the survey itself increased their interest in learning more about AIDS. Overall, these results indicate a very high interest level on the part of the respondents.

Respondents in the 1990 surveys appeared more tolerant of people with AIDS than those in the 1988 surveys. Compared to 1988, respondents in 1990 were less likely to report they would avoid contact with homosexuals for fear of contracting AIDS (50.2% in 1988; 41.4% in 1990) and more likely to support AIDS patients living at home (48.0% in 1988; 55.1% in 1990).

The respondents were classified as urban or rural residents, with the urban category including the four counties containing the major metropolitan areas in Alabama. Both of the telephone samples and the 1990 written sample could be categorized in this way, yielding 1,178 urban respondents and 1,302 rural respondents. Rural respondents in all three samples were less knowledgeable about AIDS than were urban respondents (56.3% and 59.3%, respectively). Rural respondents also were more likely than urban respondents to report that they were worried about AIDS (36.5% and 27.4%, respectively), that their concern about AIDS had caused them to change their behavior (58.0% vs. 48.0%), and to show an interest in AIDS. That is, rural respondents were more likely to report they would be willing to attend meetings to learn more about AIDS (82.6% vs. 70.5%) and were more likely to indicate that participating in the survey increased their interest in learning more about AIDS (82.7% vs. 76.4%). Finally, rural respondents were more likely than urban respondents to report that they would avoid contact with homosexuals because of their fear of AIDS (46.2% and 40.3%, respectively). This pattern of findings–rural respondents being less knowledgeable, more concerned, more interested in learning, and less tolerant than urban respondents–is consistent with those of other studies of rural-urban differences in attitudes about AIDS (Dhooper & Royse, 1989).

DISCUSSION

The instrument utilized in these surveys was intended to measure several aspects of knowledge, attitudes, and behavior. No prevention program can be successful by improving only the knowledge related to AIDS. As described by Lloyd (1990), those designing prevention programs must be aware that information alone may not provide sufficient motivation for creating or sustaining behavior change. An individual must not only have adequate information, but also feel vulnerable, and believe that the behavioral changes advocated are feasible and effective. Therefore, both knowledge and attitudes must change before it is likely that behavior will be changed.

In most regards, knowledge about AIDS transmission was accurate and, in fact, increased from 1988 to 1990. However, a majority of respondents incorrectly believed that the spread of AIDS can be prevented by using a diaphragm during sexual intercourse. If these respondents act upon this belief, they will be putting themselves or others at risk for contracting AIDS. Based on these results, MPACT has targeted this piece of misinformation as one aspect of AIDS education which needs to be emphasized.

The MPACT program has identified youth and rural communities as being among its primary target groups. Results of the surveys reported here would support such targeting, indicating that youth are in need of greater knowledge, and rural communities seem poised for attitude change.

Adolescents (up to age 19) demonstrated the lowest level of knowledge regarding AIDS. Although AIDS cases are relatively uncommon among this age group, due at least in part to the long incubation period, providing adolescents with adequate knowledge early in life could help to foster safe sexual attitudes and choices which can prevent the spread of the virus. McGill, Smith, and Johnson (1989) also report relatively low levels of knowledge on critical prevention practices even among sexually active teenagers. Educational programs are needed to provide accurate information prior to the onset of sexual activity. As DiClemente, Zorn, and Temoshok (1986) suggest, AIDS education ideally would be provided as part of a broader plan to teach students about the entire range of communicable diseases. The emphasis on youth is, of course, the long-term key to prevention of AIDS and the correlated problems of teenage pregnancy, drug abuse, and sexually transmitted diseases. The MPACT program focuses not only on AIDS prevention, but also addresses broader social and cultural issues such as self-esteem, decision-making skills, long-range planning, and a persistent emphasis on perceiving choices and anticipating the consequences of the choices.

The rural respondents were somewhat less knowledgeable, but more concerned about AIDS and more interested in learning about AIDS, compared to urban respondents. Rural respondents also were less tolerant of homosexuals. Although the greatest number of AIDS cases have been reported in the urban centers of Alabama, an increasing number of AIDS and HIV positive cases are occurring in rural areas. The absolute numbers remain low, but rates of infection are very high among minority groups in some of these counties. Several rural counties have rates of 40-50 per 100,000 minority population (compared with a statewide rate of 32.1), and one county reaches as high as 81.2 per 100,000. Many rural counties in Alabama are without adequate health care facilities and without sufficient numbers of health care professionals. Although the urban areas of the state have a relatively wide range of primary care and support services, they are unable to provide enough outreach to the surrounding communities. HIV-infected individuals in rural areas may find that their communities are not prepared to offer services or support for their physical and emotional needs (Cleveland & Davenport, 1989). Therefore, development of community education programs and plans for comprehensive services in rural areas will become increasingly critical as the incidence of AIDS in rural communities increases. The MPACT model of training local leaders and educators to provide crucial information and to facilitate attitude and behavior change is especially suited for these circumstances. In further response to these community needs, social work practitioners need to advocate for the provision of health services to rural Alabama. Furthermore, practitioners in all fields of practice need to seek opportunities to redefine their job responsibilities and provide AIDS education and other intervention activities to their clients.

Among the urban minority communities desensitization and lack of concern may be the greatest dangers. Urban respondents generally were less worried about AIDS and reported less behavior change, although the level of knowledge was somewhat higher than for rural respondents. In urban communities, therefore, emphasis may need to be placed on increasing personal vigilance and promoting long-term behavioral changes. Therefore, within urban communities as well as in rural communities, there is a great need to create qualified AIDS counselors within community agencies and facilities that already exist, such as extension centers, health centers, schools, churches, mental health centers, substance abuse programs, and community based AIDS organizations.

Although interest in learning about AIDS was greater among the rural respondents, the overall level of interest for all respondents was quite high, with approximately 80% willing to take a blood test, 80% willing to attend a meeting to learn about AIDS, and 80% indicating that participation in the survey had increased their interest in learning about AIDS. This high degree of interest suggests that this population may be very receptive to intervention efforts. Programs and services that offer a variety of AIDS education options may be particularly effective. The MPACT program is just one example of an intervention effort that is designed for the specific needs of the African-American population in Alabama. Additional intervention efforts to address this and other vulnerable populations are needed.

While a number of changes were evident over the two years

spanned by this study, it is not possible to attribute these changes directly to MPACT programs. Throughout the media there were many sources of information about AIDS during this two-year period. An increasing amount of public attention focused on the transmission and impact of AIDS within society has ultimately resulted in a more knowledgeable citizenry. The public has benefitted from the media coverage, and with the overall increase in knowledge and information has come a greater tolerance toward people with AIDS.

Continued efforts to reach adolescents and to motivate all age groups to modify their behavior in order to reduce their risks of contracting AIDS or infecting others with the virus are essential. As with the MPACT programming, information should be developed for a variety of age groups, educational levels, and cultural backgrounds. Hochhauser (cited in Fischman, 1988) reviewed sixteen AIDS information brochures published by government and private organizations and found that the typical reading level required for comprehension was that of a college sophomore. Public education needs to be written appropriately for the educational level of youth and others with limited educational backgrounds. In addition, AIDS education should be included in school curricula and the scope of services proffered by family planning clinics should be increased to include AIDS education (McGill, Smith, & Johnson, 1989). Social workers and other professionals in educational settings and family practice clinics could be utilized as resource people to discuss and clarify written information distributed to youth (McGill et al., 1989). Working within the MPACT model, social work practitioners could develop groups within local communities to provide community education (Cleveland & Davenport, 1989). These education groups could augment written information, help to reduce homophobia, and correct misinformation regarding AIDS. The success of programs such as MPACT in Alabama will rest upon their ability to deliver programs and services to African-Americans and other minorities in a manner that reflects their own culture. In addition, the written interviews included extremely heterogenous groupings. It would be useful and important to disaggregate these data in future research.

NOTES

1. The MPACT program is funded by a grant to the Cooperative Health Manpower Education Program/Tuskegee Area Health Education Center, Inc. (CHEP/ TAHEC) from the Alabama Department of Public Health. MPACT was formerly known as the Alabama AIDS In Minorities (AIM) program. For more information, contact A. Vyann Howell, CHEP/TAHEC, Inc., Veterans Administration Medical Center, Building 9, Tuskegee, AL 36083.

2. The differences in knowledge level between the written and telephone samples must be interpreted cautiously. The conditions for completing the written surveys were somewhat uncontrolled, and it is possible that some participants may have had access to written materials such as pamphlets or brochures, or may have discussed the items with other individuals in the sites where the surveys were distributed. Nevertheless, this difference was reliable, appearing at both points in time.

REFERENCES

Centers for Disease Control. (1991, May). *HIV/AIDS surveillance report.* Atlanta, GA.

Cleveland, P. H., & Davenport, J. (1989). AIDS: A growing problem for rural communities. *Human Services in the Rural Environment, 13,* 23-29.

Dalton, H. L. (1989). AIDS in blackface. *Daedalus, 118,* 205-225.

Dhooper, S. S., & Royse, D. D. (1989). Rural attitudes about AIDS: A statewide survey. *Human Services in the Rural Environment, 13,* 17-22.

DiClemente, R. J., Zorn, J., & Temoshok, L. (1986). Adolescents and AIDS: A survey of knowledge, attitudes, and beliefs about AIDS in San Francisco. *American Journal of Public Health, 76,* 1443-1445.

Fischman, J. (1988, March). AIDS: Read all about it, if you can. *Psychology Today,* p. 16.

Kappel, S., Vogt, R. L., Brozicevic, M., & Kutzko, D. (1989). AIDS knowledge and attitudes among adults in Vermont. *Public Health Reports, 104,* 388-391.

Lloyd, G. A. (1990). AIDS and HIV: The syndrome and the virus. In *Encyclopedia of social work* (18th ed., 1990 supplement, 12-50). Silver Spring, MD: National Association of Social Workers.

McGill, L., Smith, P. B., & Johnson, T. C. (1989). AIDS: Knowledge, attitudes, and risk characteristics of teens. *Journal of Sex Education & Therapy, 15,* 30-35.

Singer, E., Rogers, T. F., & Corcoran, M. (1987). The polls–a report: AIDS. *Public Opinion Quarterly, 51,* 580-595.

Singer, E., Rogers, T. F., & Glassman, M. B. (1991). Public opinion about

AIDS before and after the 1988 U.S. government public information campaign. *Public Opinion Quarterly, 55,* 161-179.

Thornberry, O. T., & Massey, J. T. (1988). Trends in United States telephone coverage across time and subgroups. In R. M. Groves, P. B. Biemer, L. E. Lyberg, J. T. Massey, W. L. Nicholls, & J. Waksberg (Eds.), *Telephone survey methodology,* (pp. 25-50). New York: Wiley.

AIDS in the Native Hawaiian Community

Noreen Mokuau
Alyson Kau

SUMMARY. Native Hawaiians are at high risk for several health disorders and experience multiple socioeconomic problems. Infection rates for AIDS in this population are increasing and, when viewed in context of their overall poor health profile, are clearly indicators for concern. This article discusses the ramifications of AIDS in the native Hawaiian community by examining the knowledge and lifestyle practices of 26 native Hawaiians in Hawaii, and by identifying recommendations that may lead to the development of culturally responsive social services.

Native Hawaiians have been consistently overlooked in the social work literature because of their relatively small population size, geographical isolation, and stereotypic image as "carefree in paradise." Emerging information on the 211,014 native Hawaiians who reside primarily in Hawaii and California (U.S. Bureau of the Census, 1990) reveals that this population is far from "carefree," but rather, impoverished and at high risk for major health disorders (Mokuau, 1990). The Native Hawaiian Health Care Improvement Act of 1988 states:

> that the health status of native Hawaiians is far below that of other United States population groups, and that in a number of areas, the evidence is compelling that native Hawaiians constitute a population group for whom the mortality rate associated with certain diseases exceed that for other United States populations in alarming proportions. (p. 23)

Noreen Mokuau, DSW, is Associate Professor/Chair, BSW, Program. Alyson Kau, MSW, is a student at the University of Hawaii, School of Social Work, Honolulu, HI 96822.

The Act reported that the overall death rate is 34 percent higher for native Hawaiians, with higher rates for diseases of the heart (44 percent), cancer (39 percent), cerebrovascular disease (31 percent) and diabetes (222 percent).

In line with such a poor health profile, native Hawaiians are beginning to show an increase in the infection rate of Acquired Immune Syndrome (AIDS). The State of Hawaii, Department of Health, through its AIDS Surveillance Quarterly Report (1990), showed that there was a cumulative total of 597 AIDS cases, with 112 (19 percent), being of Asian and Pacific Islander ancestry. Native Hawaiians have the highest number of cases among Asian and Pacific Islanders with 43 cases. Their infection rate is 19 per 100,000, second in rank to Filipinos who have an infection rate of 22 per 100,000.

AIDS statistics for native Hawaiians may not generate immediate alarm. However, when combined with information on the population's suspected high risk susceptibility to HIV, there is cause for concern. High risk factors include a high fertility rate, a rate of illegitimate births 10 percent higher than the overall average in Hawaii (Papa Ola Lokahi, 1990), the highest teen pregnancy rate in Hawaii (Tsark and Hughes, 1987), and problems in substance abuse (Takeuchi et al., 1987). In addition, the low rates of participation of native Hawaiians in programs of health education (Tsark and Hughes, 1987) suggests that vital information on AIDS containment and prevention may not be reaching this population.

This article seeks to increase social workers' awareness of AIDS among native Hawaiians by presenting preliminary information from an exploratory study of 26 native Hawaiians in Hawaii. The study assesses participants' knowledge on AIDS and further solicits their ideas on how to make health education programs appropriate for native Hawaiians.

METHODOLOGY

Sample. Twenty-six native Hawaiians from high density native Hawaiian communities in rural Hawaii were selected through purposive sampling. Due to the sensitive nature of the subject and the general reluctance among native Hawaiians to participate in such surveys, community contact persons were utilized to identify and recruit interested participants. Nineteen females (73 percent) and seven males (27 percent), ranging in age from 18 through 69 years, with a median age of 42 years, participated in the survey. Participants tended to be highly educated with 17 (65 percent) having had post-secondary education experience.

When comparing this sample with the general population of native Hawaiians, some differences emerge. The general population of native Hawaiians has fewer females (51 percent) (U.S. Bureau of the Census, 1988), is younger (median age of 25 years) (Papa Ola Lokahi, 1990), and has less experience in post secondary education (five percent) (Mokuau and Takeuchi, 1991). There are limitations in drawing generalizations from this study to the entire population due to such differences. However, the data generated from the survey does provide preliminary information on a population in which little is known.

Instrument. The survey instrument, collected information in three areas: (1) the sociodemographic characteristics of participants, (2) participants' knowledge of AIDS, and (3) participants' ideas on how to make health education programs appropriate for the native Hawaiian population. The instrument consisted of closed-ended questions and took approximately 30 minutes to complete. The instrument was developed by using information from the literature as well as from key informant interviews with nine persons recognized for their expertise in the area of AIDS.

RESULTS

General Knowledge

In general, the participants perceived themselves as having "some" knowledge on AIDS. They were asked how much they knew about AIDS, with four possible answer choices; a lot, some, a little and nothing; four (15 percent) indicated that they knew "a lot," 13 (50 percent) said they knew "some," 8 (31 percent) related that they knew "a little," and one person (4 percent) said "nothing." Participants reported that most of their information on AIDS came from the media such as newspapers, pamphlets, brochures, television and the radio.

They were then asked specific questions assessing their knowledge on AIDS, and were asked to respond "agree," "disagree," or "don't know." The majority of participants, 19 (73 percent) responded correctly to a series of questions on: (1) the definition and consequences of AIDS, (2) the differentiation of HIV and AIDS, and (3) the containment and prevention of its spread. Four persons (16 percent) answered incorrectly and three (11 percent) responded "don't know." The majority of participants also demonstrated that they were knowledgeable about the methods of transmission of the HIV as 20 (76 percent) responded correctly to questions, 2 (9 percent) responded incorrectly, and 4 (15 percent) indicated "don't know."

Ideas on Health Education Programs

Participants were asked which settings they felt would be the most appropriate for AIDS education, from whom they would feel most comfortable receiving AIDS information, and what methods were most appropriate for the presentation of the information. Participants could select more than one response. The most frequent responses to appropriate settings for AIDS education were: (1) in small groups, such as social clubs, church groups, parent groups or school clubs (73 percent), (2) in mixed groups of both men and women (65 percent), (3) in small family groups at home (54 percent), and (4) at health clinics or doctors' offices in the neighborhood (46 percent). The methods identified as most appropriate for the dissemination of information included: (1) small group discussions (81 percent), (2) one-on-one education (62 percent), and (3) lecture presentations (54 percent). Responses to appropriate educators showed a preference for receiving information from: (1) doctors, nurses and health educators, (2) teachers, and (3) church leaders.

DISCUSSION

The importance of examining AIDS among native Hawaiians relates to their low, but increasing infection rates; suspected high susceptibility; and poor overall health profile. At this point in time, AIDS may not appear to be as devastating to native Hawaiian health as other major health disorders. Yet, low rates of participation in health education programs may exacerbate their high risk health status.

This study attempted to explore the topic of AIDS in a population in which little information is available. Emphasis was on assessing 26 native Hawaiians' knowledge of AIDS and their ideas on appropriate health education programs for native Hawaiians. In a population in which the AIDS infection rates are increasing, health education programs are vital to containment and prevention.

The majority of participants (65 percent) in this survey perceived themselves as having "some" or "a lot" of knowledge about AIDS. They demonstrated that they were knowledgeable about AIDS and HIV by responding correctly to specific questions on definition and consequences, containment and prevention (73 percent), and transmission (76 percent). The results from this study are similar to results generated in an annual state-wide survey by the State of Hawaii, Department of Health, through its Health Education Office. In the state-wide study, 72 percent of the native Hawaiians respondents perceived themselves as having "some" or "a lot" of knowledge about AIDS; and 73 percent had medium or high scores on specific knowledge questions related to transmission (State of Hawaii, Department of Health, 1988). Incorrect responses reflected a lack of knowledge on AIDS transmission pertaining to blood donation, receiving blood and saliva exchange (State of Hawaii, Department of Health, 1988). In both this preliminary study and the state-wide survey, the majority of native Hawaiians are showing themselves to be informed about AIDS. However, with a fatal disease such as AIDS, full effectiveness is warranted and is based on educating 100 percent of the population.

The participants from this study indicated that they received most of their information on AIDS from media sources. This finding is consistent with information that native Hawaiians generally do not utilize health education programs (Tsark and Hughes, 1987). Lack of participation is generally attributed to the lack of accessibility and acceptability of services to the population (Mokuau and Fong, 1991). Participation in health education programs, however, is critical in the containment and prevention of HIV and AIDS and may be the vehicle in which to educate 100 percent of the population. Participants offered ideas on how to make health education programs more acceptable and comfortable for native Hawaiians.

The setting and method of presentation most preferred by the participants for education activities on AIDS was small groups. Small groups offer increased opportunities for involvement and interaction and a more personalized approach than a classroom format. The viability of group activities in native Hawaiian culture has been identified in literature focusing on instructional strategies consonant with native Hawaiian culture (D'Amato and Tharp, 1987). Group activities emphasize cultural values related to cooperation and the collective. Expanding on group activities, participants indicated that at some point in the education process, the family should be involved.

A person's perception and sense of trust in the individual who is the educator is critical to his/her decision to participate in education. Participants in the survey preferred to receive education from "local" persons. These "local" persons are defined as persons (native Hawaiians and others) who are familiar with and sensitive to the community norms and values, and have a vested interest in the community. The sensitivity of the topic and the geographic proximity of families and communities in Hawaii places high premium on an educator who can be trusted with issues too often associated with stigma and shame.

Limitations of the Study

There are limitations in the research which need to be noted. The sample was small and selected through a purposive sampling plan which makes generalizing the results of the study questionable. Furthermore, when demographic characteristics of the sample were compared with the general population, differences emerged. Future research should be designed to address external validity and enhance the utility of research findings.

Even with these limitations, however, the study has important value. It presents information on a population which has been consistently neglected in the social work literature. Furthermore, the primary source of information for this study came from native Hawaiians. Native Hawaiians are generally reticent to participate in such studies, and consequentially, they too often have been described and analyzed by non-native Hawaiians. Finally, the preliminary data generated from this study has broad implications on how to enhance participation by native Hawaiians in health education programs. These ideas can be further explored in future research and used in the design of health education programs which native Hawaiians will potentially utilize.

REFERENCES

D'Amato, J. & Tharp, R. (1987). *Culturally compatible educational strategies: implications for native Hawaiian vocational education programs.* Honolulu: University of Hawaii, Center for Studies of Multicultural Higher Education.

Mokuau, N. (1990). The impoverishment of native Hawaiians and the social work challenge. *Health and Social Work, 15*(3), 235-242.

Mokuau, N. & Fong, R. (1991). *Assessing the Responsiveness of Health Services to Ethnic Minorities of Color.* Manuscript submitted for publication.

Mokuau, N. & Takeuchi, D. T. (1991). *Leaks in the pipeline: Education among native Hawaiians.* Manuscript submitted for publication.

Native Hawaiian Health Care Improvement Act of 1988. Public Law 100-579.

Papa Ola Lokahi. (1990). *State of Hawaii Native Hawaiian health data book.* Honolulu: Office of Hawaiian Affairs.

State of Hawaii, Department of Health. (1990). *AIDS surveillance quarterly report.* Honolulu: Author.

State of Hawaii, Department of Health. (1988). *Behavioral risk factor survey.* Honolulu: Author.

Takeuchi, D. T., Higginbotham, N., Marsella, A., Gomes, K., Kwan, Jr., L., Ostrowski, B., Rocha, B. A., & Wight, K. (1987). Native Hawaiian mental health. In A. Robillard and A. Marsella (Eds.), *Contemporary issues in mental health research in the Pacific islands.* Honolulu: University of Hawaii, Social Science Research Institute.

Tsark, J. & Hughes, C. (1987). *E Ola Mau, AIDS prevention for native Hawaiians (grant proposal).* Honolulu: E Ola Mau, Inc.

U.S. Bureau of the Census. (1988). *We, the Asian and Pacific Islander Americans.* Washington, D.C.: U.S. Government Printing Office.

U.S. Bureau of the Census. (1990). *Race-Asian or Pacific Islander categories* (Summary Tape file 1A). Washington, D.C.: Author.

AIDS Prevention in a Rural Native American Population: An Empirical Approach to Program Development

Elizabeth DePoy
Claire Bolduc

SUMMARY. Currently, the primary form of AIDS prevention is behavioral. Therefore, social workers must anchor preventive efforts on empirical knowledge of the beliefs, attitudes and behavioral norms of the target reference group. This paper presents the development and implementation of a preventive social work intervention project in a rural Native American population in Maine. In order to gain an understanding of the needs of the target group, a pilot study was conducted. Based on the findings of the study, which are presented herein, and knowledge of the cultural norms of the population, a prevention program was implemented. A discussion of implications for multicultural social work practice aimed at AIDS prevention concludes the article.

INTRODUCTION

Within one short decade, AIDS has become one of the most serious health and social problems in the world (Haverekos and

Elizabeth DePoy, PhD, MSW, is Assistant Professor at the University of Maine Department of Social Work, 103 Annex C, Orono, ME 04469. Claire Bolduc, MA, is AIDS Program Director at Central Maine Indian Association, 157 Park St., Bangor, ME 04401.

Address correspondence to Elizabeth DePoy, PhD, at above address.

This project was funded by U.S. Office of Minority Health, U.S. Department of Health and Human Services–HIV Education-Prevention Grant Award.

51

Edelman, 1988; Doyle, 1988). As AIDS continues to seriously affect all groups of people, many efforts have been undertaken by social workers to prevent transmission (Cournas et al., 1989). Unfortunately, the only preventive mechanisms available at the current time are behavioral (Stall, Coates and Hoff, 1988), limiting social work intervention strategies to those which effect behavior change. Theoretically, a reduction in AIDS would follow from educating persons about the modes of transmission and reinforcing abstinence from behavior that places people at risk for contracting HIV. However, even though major educational efforts have been conducted, the incidence of AIDS continues to increase. Several studies have suggested that educational efforts may not be effective in promoting behavioral change when these efforts are not compatible with the cultural norms, level of knowledge, and patterns of behavior of the diverse reference groups receiving the educational intervention (Des Jarlais and Friedman, 1988; Hall, 1988; Fisher, 1988). The implications of studies such as those conducted by Des Jarlais and Friedman (1988) highlight the importance for social workers to practice from a culturally sensitive perspective when planning AIDS prevention and intervention for diverse ethnic, racial and cultural groups.

This paper presents a social work program in which AIDS prevention was implemented in a rural Native American community in the state of Maine. In the recognition that the Native American community holds customs and cultural norms different from those in which prevention programs previously have been conducted and documented, the program planners aimed to obtain foundation knowledge about AIDS related knowledge, attitudes and behaviors held by population members as a basis for developing an intervention tailored to the needs and norms of the Native American population in Maine.

This article presents the exploratory survey study and the AIDS prevention program which was based on a synthesis of the results of the study with relevant Native American customs.

LITERATURE REVIEW

Since the first documented case of AIDS in 1981, (CDC, 1988), the incidence of AIDS has doubled approximately every 8-10 months, creating a social and health problem of epidemic proportion (Batchelor, 1988). An overview of the literature and research on AIDS transmission and prevention reveals that infection with the AIDS virus is a result of behavior, not of group belongingness or serendipitous events (Doyle, 1988; Des Jarlais and Friedman, 1988; Peterson and Marin, 1988; Stall, Coates and Hoff, 1988; Wheeler, 1989). In the absence of pharmaceutical intervention, behavior change is therefore the only prevention strategy currently available.

Many efforts aimed at reducing behaviors which place an individual at risk for contracting the AIDS virus (herein termed AIDS risk behaviors or ARB) have been initiated since the realization that AIDS has reached epidemic proportions. The majority of these efforts involve disseminating information about AIDS transmission and prevention to those at risk (Wheeler, 1989). However, research reveals equivocal findings regarding the extent to which information acquisition promotes preventive behavior. While McKusic et al. (1985) found that sexual activity in a sample of gay men in San Francisco was not related to knowledge of AIDS risk behavior, Morin (1988) revealed a decline in risk behavior in gay men following their exposure to AIDS information. However, neither study was able to identify the factors which could predict behavior change, although both studies acknowledged that reference group norms were important to investigate further. Des Jarlais and Friedman (1988) suggest that significant factors in the presence and continuation of ARB in a reference group include the behavioral norms and knowledge held by the group members. Interestingly, even though AIDS is a major health and social problem in some minority groups, there is limited literature currently discussing prevention programs which were designed to fit with the cultural norms of those groups. The evidence pointing to the cultural group norms and beliefs as important influences on ARB suggests that social workers need to incorporate knowledge of culturally specific beliefs, norms and behaviors into their planning and implementation. Culturally relevant interventions which aim at behavior change must be developed if social workers are to be effective in promoting the reduction of ARB in culturally diverse groups.

In Maine, a predominantly rural state, there are approximately 4500 off-reservation Indians and 1300 on-reservation residents. In the summer months, the Indian population increases with the influx of migrant Indian blueberry pickers. According to informants from a local agency serving the Native American population, the Indian population holds cultural norms and customs which differ significantly from other populations in which AIDS prevention programs have been implemented. The special customs and structure of Indian society need to be understood by service providers in order to select prevention strategies which will be meaningful and credible in the Indian culture. For example, the elders hold a revered position within the Indian communities and function as transmitters of values to Indian youth (Central Maine Indian Association, 1990). This line of value transition implies that elders should be an integral part of any prevention program which is founded on behavioral change related to values.

According to Red Horse (1988), many American Indians hold beliefs about health which are inconsistent with the medical model that has served as the foundation of most AIDS education and prevention efforts. ". . . the concept of health includes a sense of harmony among sociological structures and spiritual forces"(Red Horse, 1988, p. 97). Family structures, social roles in small rural communities and gender roles are also factors which require understanding, before a meaningful prevention program can be planned. Red Horse (1988) indicates that rural Indian families tend to exhibit traditional gender roles and maintain a closed community.

Unfortunately, the incidence of AIDS is increasing in the total Indian population in Maine. Currently, there are twelve reported cases of AIDS, multiple cases of HIV infection and it is estimated that the majority of cases of AIDS and HIV infection in the Indian population in Maine are unreported (Central Maine Indian Association Report, 1989). According to informants from the CMIA (Central Maine Indian Association), the major form of HIV transmission in the Indian culture is through unprotected sex. Reportedly, the predominant drug abused in the Indian culture in Maine is alcohol. The combination of unprotected sex with multiple partners and alcohol abuse has been shown to be a major risk in AIDS behavior in other populations (Stall, 1988). With the risk factors present and the incidence of AIDS increasing at alarming rates, the need to establish prevention programs is paramount. However, to insure the likelihood of decreasing the spread of AIDS, these programs must be empirically anchored on the knowledge, behaviors and norms of the Native American population to whom the prevention effort is directed.

THE STUDY

The purpose of the study was to obtain information about the knowledge, attitudes, and risk behaviors related to AIDS in the target Native American reference group, as a basis for developing a culturally relevant AIDS prevention intervention.

The following four research questions were answered by the study:

1. What is the level of knowledge held by the Indian population in Maine about AIDS transmission, AIDS symptoms and the disease process?
2. What attitudes about AIDS and persons with AIDS are held by the Indian population in Maine?
3. What is the level of AIDS risk behavior in the Indian population in Maine?
4. What is the relationship among level of knowledge, attitudes and ARB in this population?

A two member team, consisting of a social worker and a service provider in an agency that serves the Indian population planned and conducted the research. Each member brought essential expertise to the study. The primary investigator (the service provider) was able to insure that design and instrumentation were consistent with cultural boundaries in the Indian community and that questions were framed to reflect the culture of the participating Indian communities. The co-investigator, a social work educator, provided the research design expertise. In order to maintain confidentiality of respondents, particularly in light of the sensitive nature of the inquiry (Melton and Gray, 1988), the team selected a survey approach to answer the research questions.

Sample

The non-random sample was recruited by the researchers and the tribal staff who served as research assistants at four different tribal centers over a three month period of time. The tribal centers are locations where community members gather for social, political and other community events. One hundred and seventy subjects were available to participate in the project. All subjects were Indians who resided in the state of Maine at the time of the study. All but nine of the subjects belonged to the Passamaquody tribe. Although the research assistants attempted to restrict participation to adults, surveys were distributed, self administered and collected from all willing participants for the purpose of confidentiality. Not all respondents answered all questions. A total of 154 questionnaires were completed sufficiently for data analysis and were used as the sample responses. Table 1 describes the demographic characteristics and tribal affiliations of the sample.

Instrumentation

A questionnaire was developed by the research team to elicit information in four categories: Category A–demographic information, including age, gender, and marital status; Category B–knowledge of AIDS transmission, symptom recognition and disease process; Category C–attitudes towards contracting HIV and towards persons with AIDS; and Category D–frequency of ARB. Categories were not identified to the respondents, but rather used in data analysis. The content and structure of the questionnaire were developed by the primary investigator and co-investigator. The questionnaire was then pilot tested by three researchers and two lay respondents and revised in response to pilot test findings. The team was careful to use culturally sensitive language at a reading level consistent with the documented minimum reading skills of the population. In addition, the questionnaire was limited to 7 minutes of response time in order to increase the participation rate of potential subjects. The content of the questionnaire included items, such as potential transmission of HIV through eating non-domesticated animal meat such as moose, that reflect the lifestyle, customs and common sense beliefs of the target population.

TABLE 1. Demographic Characteristics and Tribal Affiliation
(n = 154)

	Frequency	%
Tribal Affiliation		
Penobscot	4	2.6
Passamaquody	143	94.1
Micmac	3	2.0
Other	2	1.3
Unknown	2	1.3
Age		
under 19	19	12.2
20-29	46	29.8
30-39	49	32.0
40-49	17	11.0
50-59	7	5.0
60+	16	10.0
Gender		
Male	52	33.8
Female	102	66.2

In section A, demographic data were collected. Section B, on knowledge, contained 27 true-false items on AIDS transmission, prevention and disease recognition and process, also yielding an interval level score of the number of correct responses. Eleven true-false items comprised Section C, on attitudes, and four multiple choice items were contained in *Section D*, on ARB. In *Section C*, the range of scores, 0-11, indicated conservative-liberal attitudes respectively. (Conservative attitudes were operationalized as those which demonstrated less tolerance for persons with AIDS and for risk behavior. Liberal scores were operationalized as those responses which demonstrated more tolerance for persons with AIDS and for risk behaviors. The liberal-conservative structure was used for data analysis only and is not intended to imply value judgement.) On *Section D*, the range was 4-12, creating a scale of low to high risk behaviors respectively. Because the study was a needs assessment that was limited in time by funding constraints, no reliability and validity studies were completed on the instrumentation.

Procedures

At four separate time intervals, questionnaires were administered to a total of 170 subjects. As mentioned above, due to incomplete responses to items, particularly on the demographic section, only 154 of those were included in the study. After consenting to participate, each subject was assured of confidentiality, and was given the questionnaire and an unmarked envelope. The subjects independently completed the questionnaires immediately, placed the instrument in the envelope and handed the envelope to a research assistant, who coded the contents for tribal affiliation.

Data analysis was conducted by using three statistical techniques. First, frequencies and percentages were calculated for all survey items, and group mean scores for Sections B, C, and D were calculated. ANOVA was then used to discern differences in scores related to gender. Finally, the Pearson R correlation coefficient was calculated between sections to determine if a relationship existed among knowledge, attitudes and risk behaviors. (N.B. Not all respondents answered all questions adequately to be coded as a response or missing data. In this case, the data were omitted from analysis, yielding different "frequencies" for some of the items.)

RESULTS

Knowledge

Tabular analysis of items on the knowledge section suggest that in general, the respondents were knowledgeable about AIDS transmission and symptoms. Some misconceptions, however existed, on items exploring person to person transmission. (Table 2 presents frequency data for items asking about person to person transmission.)

Respondents were also generally knowledgeable about the modes of HIV transmission. However, some incorrect responses were noted on items asking about blood and body fluid exchange. (Table 3 depicts frequency analysis for modes of transmission items.)

In the section on knowledge regarding AIDS prevention, experience of AIDS, and persons with AIDS, percentages of incorrect responses on each item ranged from 4.5% to 31.2%. The largest percentage of error was noted on the items relating to condom use as an AIDS prevention (Table 4 presents frequency analysis for items in the subcategory). Mean sample score for the total number of correct responses on the knowledge section of the questionnaire was 22.4 (SD = 4.5) out of a potential perfect score of 27, indicating a relatively high degree of knowledge.

Analysis of missing cases demonstrates high rate of non-response to several items. In methods of HIV transmission, 19 (12.3%) non-responses were calculated on the item asking if AIDS can be transmitted from woman to woman, compared to a mean of 9.8 on other questions asking about methods of HIV transmission. Higher non-response rates (n = 16, n = 13) were noted on questions asking if AIDS was transmitted by sweat and tears respectively. Twelve non-responses (7.8%) were noted when respondents were asked if they could get AIDS.

ANOVA was conducted to determine gender differences on each section. On the knowledge section, the male group scores indicated

TABLE 2. Transmission from Person to Person

	frequency			%			
	correct	incorrect	missing	correct	incorrect	missing	n
man to man	138	6	10	89.6	3.9	6.5	154
woman to woman	116	19	19	75.3	12.3	12.3	154
man to woman	136	9	9	88.3	5.8	5.8	154
woman to unborn child	137	8	9	89.0	5.2	5.8	154

TABLE 3. Modes of Transmission

item	correct	frequency incorrect	missing	percent correct	incorrect	missing	n
sex	144	6	4	93.5	4.0	2.6	154
toilet seats	131	14	9	85.1	9.0	5.9	154
kissing	115	29	10	74.7	18.8	6.5	154
sharing utensils	123	21	10	79.9	13.6	6.5	154
hugging	142	2	10	92.2	1.3	6.5	154
touching	137	8	9	89.0	5.8	5.2	154
bug bites	122	23	9	79.2	14.9	5.9	154
black flies	127	17	10	82.5	11.0	6.6	154
deer meat	134	8	12	87.0	5.2	7.8	154
moose meat	136	7	11	88.3	4.5	7.2	154
tears	122	19	13	79.2	12.3	8.5	154
sweat	114	24	16	74.0	15.6	10.4	154
sharing needles	142	6	6	92.2	3.9	3.9	154
giving blood	100	41	3	64.9	26.6	1.9	154
receiving blood	133	18	3	86.4	11.7	1.9	154

TABLE 4. Prevention

item	frequency			%			n
	correct	incorrect	missing	correct	incorrect	missing	
I can't get AIDS	129	13	12	83.8	8.4	7.8	154
Condoms can protect during oral sex	98	48	8	63.6	31.2	5.2	154
Condoms can protect during anal sex	120	26	8	77.9	16.9	5.2	154
Condoms can protect during vaginal sex	127	22	5	82.5	14.3	3.2	

significantly more dispersion and lower scores than women's scores. Mean scores and standard deviations were 22.6 and 3.9514 respectively for females and 22.46 and 5.8268 respectively for males (F $(1,152)$ = 8.2989, p = .0004).

Attitudes

Scores on attitude items varied on the liberal conservative scale. The items which received the most conservative responses were those relating to willingness to care for persons with AIDS. More liberal responses were demonstrated on questions asking for moral judgement of persons with AIDS. (For example, one item examining moral judgements about PWAs was worded as "People who have AIDS are bad people.") Items about isolating or punishing persons with AIDS received consensus from 87% of the respondents that neither children or adults should be excluded from mainstream society.

Mean score for the total sample was 8.7(SD = 2.0).

ANOVA revealed that males scored significantly lower (more conservative) than females at p = .0486. Mean scores and standard deviations were 8.3077 and 1.8528 respectively for males and 8.93 and 1.9019 respectively for females (F$(1,152)$ = 3.9532, p = .0486).

Risk Behavior

Mean score for the total sample on the section testing AIDS risk behavior was 6.6 on a scale from 4-12, indicating a relatively low degree of overall risk behavior. Risk behavior was determined by the frequency of sexual relations with unfamiliar partners, the frequency of condom use and the extent to which subjects reported that they were concerned about contracting the HIV virus. The greatest risk behavior of contracting AIDS was in the area of condom use. Sixty-one percent of the respondents reported that they never used condoms (a high risk behavior) and 26% reported that they use condoms only sometimes (a moderate risk behavior). Almost 10% report that they have had sex in the past year with persons who they did not know. ANOVA revealed that males (mean score = 6.19, SD = 1.2214) demonstrate significantly lower risk behavior than females (mean score = 6.79, SD = 1.1308) (F (1, 152) = 5.26, p = .0062).

Relationship Among Knowledge, Attitudes and Behaviors

The Pearson R correlation coefficient was calculated to determine if relationships existed between any two of the three sections. The only significant correlation was noted between knowledge and attitudes (r = .6123, p = ≤ .005). However, in this sample, level of AIDS risk behavior was not significantly related to either knowledge or attitudes.

DISCUSSION

Before interpreting the findings, two limitations in the study design need to be noted. First, the study is exploratory and uses a non-random sample. The volunteer nature of the sample may affect internal and external validity. Second, the sample is heavily weighted towards one tribal group, thereby indicating caution when considering external validity and the ability of the study to reveal distinctions in the knowledge, attitudes and risk behaviors of persons from differing tribal affiliations.

The data analysis suggests many tenets about AIDS knowledge, attitudes and risk behavior in the sample. First, the level of knowledge about HIV transmission, prevention and experience is generally high, suggesting that the population is generally knowledgeable about HIV transmission and experience. However, three areas of misconception seem to exist. First, while medical experts insist that AIDS is only transmitted through blood exchange and sexual activity (Doyle, 1988), a high percentage of respondents indicated that they believe that the HIV virus can be spread through other body fluids either by direct contact or by insect and animal carrier. The causes of these misconceptions warrant further study as a basis for the establishment of relevant and believable prevention programs. Second, questions about the extent to which women could transmit or receive the HIV virus revealed a high degree of uncertainty. Third, responses to questions about condom use suggested that a large percentage of respondents many not have viewed condoms as a reliable means of protection or saw no reason to use them.

The correct responses on the knowledge section seem to reflect stereotypical notions (Des Jarlais and Freidman, 1988) of who can get AIDS and how it is transmitted, raising questions on what sources of knowledge are believed. Areas of misconception may be linked not to expert opinion, but rather to culturally specific and socially accepted belief. It seems as if people are very aware of AIDS, are talking about it, but may not be accepting expert opinion regarding mode of transmission.

The section on attitudes suggests that while persons are becoming more accepting of AIDS, a high percentage would not consider becoming caretakers of family members or friends who have AIDS. In order to determine the reasons for relinquishing these social responsibilities, further investigation should be initiated, particularly in light of the increasing financial, social, and psychological cost of institutionalization.

Findings related to AIDS risk behaviors suggest that risk behavior is relatively low in most areas. However, one area, that of condom use, is particularly noteworthy. In light of the misconceptions about the value of condoms in AIDS prevention demonstrated in the knowledge section, it is not surprising that condom use is so sporadic. Further, because women seemed to exhibit significantly higher risk behaviors than the male subjects through unprotected sex, the low frequency of condom use may be a result of the traditional gender roles of women in the Native American culture (Red Horse, 1988) in that women may not perceive themselves as the responsible party for AIDS protection or for contraception. However, because IV drug use is not a major method of HIV transmission in the Indian population (Central Maine Indian Association, 1989), risk seems to loom in the behavior of unprotected sex.

In addition to the descriptive findings discussed above, two major relational findings are important. The gender differences in all three areas of knowledge, attitudes and behaviors are notable. Male respondents tend to hold less accurate knowledge, and more conservative beliefs about AIDS and persons with AIDS, suggesting different social norms for each gender. A second and critical finding is in the relationship among knowledge, attitudes and behaviors. While knowledge and attitudes are positively related, that is to say, more accurate knowledge is related to more liberal attitudes, there is not a significant correlation between risk behavior and either knowledge or attitudes. This complex relationship in the Native American population seems to be consistent with previous studies (Des Jarlais and Friedman, 1988) and suggested very important findings for AIDS prevention in the sample that was tested in this study.

THE PREVENTION PROGRAM

The study revealed important findings upon which prevention strategies were then anchored. First, the knowledge of AIDS and HIV in the respondent group was generally high, speaking to the success of general prevention efforts and thereby eliminating the need for major educational efforts. However, in spite of a generally high degree of knowledge, risk factors still exist in the Native American population that were identified through the study. The three basic areas for prevention include: (1) HIV transmission, (2) transmission between genders, and (3) sexual prevention strategies, with particular attention to women's issues and gender norms.

Education and prevention around the above three areas were accomplished through interventions which were developed by members of the Native American community. Because the findings in the study revealed that unprotected sex was a major area of risk for the Indian population, a major emphasis was placed on safe sex. In an effort to encourage more women to consider condom use, condom jewelry, fabricated by an Indian to display traditional Indian design was distributed. Second, consistent with elders' role (Red Horse, 1988), respected elders in the community were recruited to discuss safe sex with the youth. To address other areas of knowledge, attitudes and beliefs about HIV and persons with AIDS, a theater troupe was commissioned to stage a series of plays, following which discussion and reaction to the material presented would take place and be facilitated by a respected member of the community. The theater was selected as a culturally valued medium for presentation of sensitive issues. The scripts will include information on HIV transmission, vignettes aimed at understanding the experience of AIDS and messages about the responsibility of both genders to exercise safe sex. The discussion groups will be aimed at re-education around misconceptions, feelings about health and wellness related to AIDS and about values and prevention that fit with the cultural norms.

Each of these prevention interventions will be fully evaluated in the future to determine the extent to which risk behavior was reduced.

BROADER PRACTICE IMPLICATIONS

Based on literature and the findings of the pilot project, it seems likely that beliefs about HIV transmission may be a cultural phenomenon, in part determined by myth and common knowledge (Red Horse, 1988). The extent to which medical sources are believed by various cultures needs further exploration. Further research should examine the sources for inaccurate knowledge as a basis for identifying the culturally relevant vehicles through which knowledge can be disseminated and more importantly, believed. Once the socially and culturally accepted methods of changing knowledge and beliefs are understood in target groups, relevant and meaningful methods can be used by social workers to transmit accurate AIDS prevention information (Des Jarlais and Friedman, 1988).

Furthermore, it is even more important to note that accurate knowledge and liberal attitudes towards AIDS may be necessary but insufficient, by themselves, for behavior change. Therefore, interventions need to move beyond offering only knowledge. Social workers must discover the social and cultural factors which promote risk behavior. Only then can they plan strategies which elicit change. AIDS prevention, therefore, must be examined and treated not only as a health problem but as a social-cultural phenomenon.

Finally, this study illuminates the importance of social work research as a prerequisite to the development of preventive interventions in general. It is clear that AIDS prevention is not a unitary strategy in any culture, but needs to be carefully planned to be relevant to the beliefs, norms and demonstrated behaviors of the population to which the efforts are directed.

REFERENCES

Batchelor, W. (1988) AIDS 1988, the science and the limits of science. *American Psychologist, 11,* 853-858.

Centers for Disease Control. (1988) *AIDS weekly surveillance report-United States.* April 11.

Coates, T., Stall, R., Kegeles, S., Lo, B., McKusick, L. (1988) AIDS antibody testing, will it stop the AIDS epidemic? Will it help people infected with HIV? *American Psychologist, 11,* 859-861.

Cournas, F., Empfield, M., Horwath, E., Kramer, M. (1989) The management of HIV infection in state psychiatry hospitals. *Hospital and Community Psychiatry, 2,* 153-157.

Des Jarlais, D., and Friedman, S. (1988) The psychology of preventing AIDS among intravenous drug users, a social learning conceptualization. *American Psychologist, 11,* 865-870.

Doyle, D. (1988)The meaning of AIDS. *Commonwealth,* June 3, 115.

Fisher, J. (1988) Possible effects of reference group-based social influence on AIDS risk behavior and AIDS prevention. *American Psychologist, 11,* 914-920.

Hall, L. (1988) Social work update: Providing culturally relevant mental health services for central American immigrants. *Hospital and Community Psychiatry, 11,* 1139-1144.

Haney, P. (1988) Providing empowerment to persons with AIDS. *Social Work, 33,* 251-253.

Haverekos, H. and Edelman, R. (1988) The epidemiology of AIDS among heterosexuals. *The Journal of the American Medical Association, 7,* 260.

Mann, J. (1989) AIDS and discrimination. *World Health,* June 3.

Meinhardt, K. and Vegg, W. (1987) A method for establishing underutilization of mental health services by ethnic groups. *Hospital and Community Psychiatry, 11,* 1186-1190.

Morin, S. (1988) AIDS: the challenge to psychology. *American Psychologist, 11,* 838-842.

Perry, S. and Mancowitz, J. (1988) Counseling for HIV testing. *Hospital and Community Psychiatry, 7,* 731-737.

Peterson, J. and Marin, G. (1988) Issues in the prevention of AIDS among black and hispanic men. *American Psychologist, 11,* 871-877.

Quinn, T., Zacarias, F., and St. John, R. (1989) AIDS in the Americas: An emerging public health crisis. *New England Journal of Medicine, 23,* 320.

Red Horse, J. (1988) in Jacobs, C. and Bowles, D., eds. Ethnicity and race: *Critical concepts in social work.* Silver Springs, MD: NASW.

Rounds, K. (1988) AIDS in rural areas: Challenges to providing care. *Social Work, 33,* 257-261.

Stall, R., Coates, T., Hoff, C. (1988) Behavior risk reduction for HIV among gay and bisexual men. *American Psychologist, 11,* 878-885.

Weiss, R. (1988) New models for AIDS in third world countries. *Science News,* March 19, 133.

Wheeler, D. (1989) New studies urged on cultural factors in spread of AIDS. *The Chronicle of Higher Education,* June 14.

A Survey of AIDS Knowledge and Attitudes Among Prostitutes in an International Border Community

Felipe Peralta
Patricia A. Sandau-Beckler
Rosario H. Torres

SUMMARY. Prostitutes are a *high risk population* engaged in high risk behavior for the transmission of HIV Disease (AIDS). This paper presents the results of a survey to evaluate the knowledge, attitudes and behaviors of prostitutes about HIV Disease (AIDS). This survey was conducted in an International Border Community. A total of sixty women participated in this survey. The sources of information on AIDS and its accuracy were explored. The impact of this knowledge on behavior was identified. The most important finding is that the prostitutes are not utilizing risk reduction behaviors while having sexual relations with their clients. The survey found that fifty-four percent of the participants did not use condoms on a regular basis. And an alarming ten percent did not use condoms at all. The results of this survey have implications for social workers and public health workers who must develop strategies to work effectively with this high risk population.

Felipe Peralta, MSW, is Assistant Professor and Patricia A. Sandau-Beckler, ACSW, is Assistant Professor at the Department of Social Work, New Mexico State University, Las Cruces, NM 88003-0001. Rosario H. Torres, CSW-ACP, ACSW, is Director of Social Services and HIV Project Coordinator at Centro de Salud Familiar La Fe, Inc., 700 S. Ochoa, El Paso, TX 79901.

This survey was partially supported by the Deans Research Funds, New Mexico State University.

INTRODUCTION

Not since diseases like the bubonic plague, which killed 17 to 18 million people, one-third of Europe's population, has an epidemic had the potential global impact of AIDS. The World Health Organization predicts that up to 30 million people will die from the human immunodeficiency virus (HIV) in the next decade (Heise, 1988). This issue particularly affects lesser developed countries.

This paper is a review of a survey of a population group engaged in behavior which is considered risky for the transmission of the AIDS virus. A group of prostitutes was surveyed in the international border communities of El Paso, Texas, and Ciudad (Cd.) Juarez, Chihuahua, Mexico. The participants live and work in Cd. Juarez. Their clients are from both Mexico and the United States.

The researchers asked about the knowledge this population group has about the transmission of HIV, their frequency in using risk reduction techniques, the implications for their own health, that of their families and clients, and for the further spread of the disease. This paper is a summary of survey results and the implications for education and prevention efforts in international border communities.

REVIEW OF THE LITERATURE

One of the difficulties in understanding the implications of AIDS is society's negative attitudes toward populations identified as engaging in high risk behaviors. This creates the development of "underground" subsystems, making evaluation of such groups difficult. This is particularly true for prostitutes (Jaget, 1980; Perkins & Bennett, 1985; and Delacoste & Alexander, 1987).

The International Problem of Prostitution and the Spread of AIDS

Public health officials worldwide have targeted prostitutes as a group whose behavior puts them at high risk of contracting and spreading the HIV. Johnson (1988, p. 1017) noted "little incidence of HIV infection in European prostitutes (from one to ten percent), except for those involved in IV drug use.'' In Africa, where HIV infection is associated with heterosexual activities (Kreiss et al., 1986), infection among prostitutes ranges from 26 percent in Zaire to 82 percent in Rwanda (Plant et al., 1989). This study is an attempt to participate in the creation of a body of knowledge concerning the United States-Mexico border and the generalizability of the findings to prostitutes and HIV/AIDS infection. The authors were unable to find any other studies examining knowledge and attitudes among prostitutes on the United States-Mexican border.

Global Barriers to Research on Effectiveness of Prevention Education for AIDS with Prostitutes

Numerous factors hamper research on the effectiveness of prevention education.

The first factor is the moral and sexist attitudes surrounding the business of prostitution, which serve to curtail research about prostitutes, a minority group routinely used as a scapegoat in this and other countries. Self-deprecation by prostitutes and a lack of trust that prevents them from seeking health services and health education are additional factors. At times prostitutes may see themselves as not entitled to these services. Furthermore, they may distrust the government's motives for helping them, fearing punishment if they identify themselves or their behaviors.

Additionally, governmental denial of the presence of the disease, and the economic impact of responding to the needs for AIDS education adversely impact prevention efforts. Public health campaigns about AIDS education in some countries ''means diverting scarce or non-existent resources into what may be a non-economic venture'' (Shaw, 1987, p. 20).

Equally important may be governments ignoring the reasons and conditions that perpetuate prostitution within their countries. Prostitution is often a means of making a living and supporting one's family. Women with minimal job entry skills, who have been ejected from their families because of early pregnancy, or who have drug habits, may view prostitution as their only means of support.

Cultural differences also contribute to the lack of effective AIDS research and prevention. This includes embarrassment about discussing sexual matters openly and denial in recognizing the possibility that trusted family members could be involved in risky behavior. In some cultures, women's role preclude their asking partners to use condoms; condom use may threaten the implied trust within the relationship. Prostitutes tend not to use condoms with their husbands or significant others, many of whom may be at high risk for HIV and other Sexually Transmitted Diseases (STD's) (Rosenberg & Weiner, 1988).

Studies of Knowledge, Attitudes, and Behaviors

The few studies available on knowledge, attitudes, and behaviors of prostitutes in developing nations show cause for much concern. For example, a study in Borno, Nigeria indicated that even after education, of 764 prostitutes interviewed, only 77.1 percent recalled that the use of condoms during sex reduced the risk of spreading the disease. When assessing the knowledge of transmission modes only 75.7% knew that sexual intercourse transmitted the virus. "Some (8.6%), however, mentioned kissing and other casual contacts as potential modes of transmission of the virus" (Chikwem et al., 1988, page 443). The study concluded that a continuation of vigorous health education and prevention methods is necessary for prostitutes who are unlikely to discontinue their risky behavior because of the financial necessity to support themselves and their dependents through prostitution.

A wide range of behavioral responses to using condoms has been noted worldwide. The following studies reflect the great diversity of responses. A study of prostitutes in Santo Domingo indicated that only one-third of the women studied confirmed they used condoms with their last customer (Pareja, Rosario, Smith, Butler de Lister & Guerrero, 1989). In a study in Singapore, of one hundred prostitutes, "half of the 59 women who were not using diaphragms nor antibiotics indicated that between a quarter and a half of their clients used condoms and a quarter said that fewer than a quarter of their clients used condoms" (Bradbeer, Thin, Tan, & Thirumoorthy, 1987, p. 52). Studies done in Zaire with 377 prostitutes indicated the low use of condoms, with prostitutes reporting using condoms less than half the time (Mann et al., 1988). In England, a study of prostitutes indicated that 62% always used condoms with 6.1% indicating that they never use condoms (Thomas, Plant, Plant, Sales, 1989).

In a San Francisco study, J.B. Cohen and Coweeks (1989) found that "90% of prostitutes reported at least one instance of condom use with paying clients" and that "38% said they always used condoms with clients, compared to only 14% who sometimes used condoms with husbands or boyfriends" (Miller, Turner & Moses, 1990). This contrasts with a group of prostitutes studied in Birmingham where the condom use rate was 90% (Plant, Plant, Peck & Setters, 1989). As a result of education done in Nairobi, Monlase, and Kenya prostitutes demonstrate less willingness to engage in sexual contact with customers who refuse to wear condoms (Alexander, 1988). Another approach to condom use might be education directed towards men who refuse the use of condoms (Alexander, 1988). In Germany prostitutes are proposing that laws be passed to mandate condom use (Alexander, 1988).

Another issue for prostitutes and their behavior in relation to HIV is that they are "less likely to use condoms with their husbands or boyfriends than with clients" (Darrow, 1990, p. 16). This puts them at greatest risk of contracting HIV virus from their husbands, boyfriends or significant others (Rosenberg & Weiner, 1988).

In order to understand the attitudes and behaviors of prostitutes in the international border communities located along the 2,000 miles of border the United States shares with Mexico, attention should be given to people of Mexican ancestry. Information about their cultural attitudes and knowledge about AIDS is important in developing research strategies, education, and prevention methods. A National Health Review survey, published in 1989 and sponsored by the Centers for Disease Control, explored Hispanic Americans' attitudes and knowledge about AIDS (Dawson & Hardy, 1989). Persons of Mexican ancestry were defined as a subgroup in this survey. They faired poorly on accurate knowledge about transmission of AIDS. Communication about the subject indicated a lack of trust in government information and advice (Dawson & Hardy, 1989).

INTERNATIONAL SURVEY OF PROSTITUTES IN A BORDER COMMUNITY

During the Spring of 1990, a survey to evaluate the knowledge, attitudes, and behaviors of prostitutes about AIDS was conducted at the San Felipe Women's Clinic in Ciudad Juarez. The following is a description of the setting, background, and the results of this survey.

The International Setting. El Paso, Texas, population about 600,000, is a major gateway to Mexico via Cd. Juarez, population approximately 1.4 million. About 40 million people cross between the two cities annually, making it the second largest port of entry to the United States.

El Paso's population is primarily Mexican-American (66 percent). The city's per capita income is nearly 30 percent lower than the national average; more than one-fifth of the city's population falls below the national poverty level. The close proximity and high mobility of the two cities' populations have a marked impact on the health care and human services systems in both communities.

It is estimated that Cd. Juarez has approximately 5,000 prostitutes, while El Paso has about 1,000 (El Paso The City-County Health District, 1990). El Paso also has approximately 9,000 heroin addicts (Aliviane NO-AD, Inc.). Of these addicts, a significant number are women who engage in prostitution as a means of supporting their addictions.

Several widely recognized prostitution zones exist in both cities, with prostitutes intermingling between cities (it is a five to ten-minute walk between the two downtown areas). Analysis of STD/HIV cases demonstrates that persons having regular as well as occasional contact with prostitutes are consistently low in use of condoms. The above factors point to the need for further research and analysis of knowledge, attitude, and behavior patterns of prostitutes in the two communities. Mexico has a National Center for AIDS Information which provides education for prostitutes. They advocate direct contact with prostitutes in their own communities (Alexander, 1988).

Survey and Methodology

The survey was conducted at the San Felipe Women's Clinic located four miles from downtown Ciudad Juarez. This clinic has been in operation for fifteen years and is funded and operated by the federal government. San Felipe Clinic provides obstetric and gynecological medical services at low cost to all women in this community. There are about 400 women who are involved in prostitution who receive their medical care at this clinic. These women are tested for HIV and other communicable diseases. The clinic facility is also utilized for educational meetings for the women who come for medical services.

Each participant in this survey was interviewed following a questionnaire consisting of 21 items. The interview questionnaires were conducted in Spanish by two bilingual, male and female, social workers holding master of social work degrees. Participants were selected on random days from women arriving at the clinic for regularly scheduled or walk-in appointments. Participation was voluntary; sixty women comprised the sample. In order to gain the respondents' trust, the clinic's medical director introduced the interviewers to the participants and explained the purpose of the survey. The interviews lasted fifty to sixty minutes.

The participants were willing and very candid in their answers which clearly reflect their behavior. The women were impressed that researchers were interested in their well being. The participants wanted more information and were interested in the development of educational groups.

RESULTS OF THE SURVEY

Characteristics of the Participants in the Survey Sample

Age. The ages of the women who participated in the survey ranged from nineteen to fifty with the average age being 29. Seventeen percent of the participants were 29 and 30 years old.

Marital Status. During the time that this study was undertaken, 53.3% of the women who participated reported being single. Another 21.7% of the women reported being divorced. The percentage of women who reported being married was 15.0. Five percent of the women reported being widowed and another 5.0% reported being separated.

Children. Only four women who participated in the survey had no biological children. Thirty-seven of the women had one or two children. Fifteen of the women reported having between three and six children. One participant had eight children and another one had ten children. Two did not answer this question.

Clients Served. Survey respondents served clients from both Mexico and the United States. Forty (66 percent) indicated that most of their clients were from Mexico; ten respondents (17 percent) identified most of their clients as being from the United States. Thirteen percent of the women said they served an equal number of clients from Mexico and the United States. Two women did not answer this question.

Sources of Information About AIDS. Respondents identified a district health clinic, television, the print media, friends, and clients as sources of information about AIDS. Significant to this study was the role the district Health Clinic played in providing information. Ninety-two percent of the women said that they received information from this source. More information and study needs to occur on the accuracy of friends' and clients' information provided to prostitutes.

Knowledge of AIDS Transmission. All of the respondents knew that AIDS could be transmitted through sexual contact. All but one knew that AIDS could be transmitted by sharing needles, and all but two knew that AIDS could be transmitted during blood transfusions. Of significance is that 40% believed that kissing and 23% believed that sharing utensils were transmission methods, clearly demonstrating a need for accurate information.

Knowledge of Risk Behaviors. Respondents identified the following activities as low-risk: massages (88 percent); vaginal sexual intercourse using a condom (75 percent); mutual masturbation (70 percent); anal intercourse using a condom (62 percent); oral sex using a condom (62 percent); oral sex not using a condom (23 percent); and vaginal sexual intercourse not using a condom (12 percent).

Beliefs About Low Risk Transmission. Thirty-two percent of the respondents reported knowing how to lower the risk of infection while sharing needles by cleaning needles with Clorox and avoiding the use of dirty needles. The high percentage of women who did not know how to lower risk while using needles for intravenous drugs may be because few participants admitted personally knowing people who used intravenous drugs.

Use of Condoms. Respondents were asked how many times they used condoms during their previous ten sexual encounters. Ten percent of the respondents did not use condoms at all and 30% used them less than one half of the time. Forty-six percent indicated using condoms during the past ten sexual encounters. Sixty-three percent reported that condom use was discussed with clients; the others did not discuss condom use with clients. Thirty-seven percent of respondents reported having sexual intercourse with clients who refused to use condoms, particularly if they knew the client. This finding is consistent with other studies where the prostitute is at risk for AIDS virus. Sixty percent of the participants reported that if a client refused to use a condom, they refused to have sexual intercourse with him.

Predicted Response to HIV Infection. Ninety-five percent of the participants reported they would undergo further testing if they suspected they were infected with HIV. Two women said they would refuse testing, one woman did not answer this question.

Respondents indicated that concern for their children's safety and obtaining medical services would be of primary importance if they tested positive for HIV. Six women said they would know what to do if they tested positive; one person said she would consider committing suicide as a potential response, and another said she would cease prostitution so as not to infect other people.

DISCUSSION

Of the estimated 6,000 prostitutes in Cd. Juarez and El Paso, seventy percent are carriers of HIV (El Paso City County Health

District, 1990). If this figure is accurate, the potential pandemic in a bi-national area of scarce health and social services for the medically indigent on both sides of the border, could become a problem of massive proportions. It is impossible to assess the psychosocial and financial price tag at this time. However, the people affected by the infection could be the general population of both sides. In general, people seeking sex from prostitutes, and crossing the border, do not think of themselves as engaging in a high risk behavior. The present survey is a first step in evaluating the knowledge, attitudes, and behaviors of prostitutes working primarily in low-income areas of Cd. Juarez in relation to the transmission of the HIV.

Of the women surveyed, forty-six percent reported using condoms on a regular basis. Compared to other studies, in particular the one by Pareja, Rosario, Smith, Butler de Lister and Guerrero (1989), this represents a low rate of condom use. Thirty-seven percent in this study continued to have sex with clients who refused to use condoms. This was consistent with other findings in Scotland (Goldberg et al., 1988; Thomas et al., 1989). An alarming ten percent did not use condoms at all. Although 94 percent of the respondents had received basic information about AIDS, its transmission, and prevention methods from a number of sources, including clients, health workers, and print and broadcast media, forty percent of them held inaccurate beliefs with regard to such things as acquiring the infection by kissing and sharing utensils.

Ninety-five percent of the respondents said they would seek testing and medical attention if they suspected being infected by the HIV. Fifty-two percent of them, however, did not know where to go for medical care. Two respondents indicated they would seek medical care in El Paso. All of the participants reported being concerned about the disease in general, and 71 percent reported that relatives or friends were concerned about the respondents' risk of contracting AIDS because of their occupation. It appears that multi-level primary prevention efforts need to be on-going. Paying close attention to the acquiring and the integrating of information is essential. In addition, if information is targeted to a "high risk group," the assumption may be generated to the rest of the population that they need not be concerned. Consequently, family education may become less probable.

IMPLICATIONS FOR PRACTICE

The results of this survey demonstrate that women who are involved in prostitution in a border setting have a limited knowledge about the AIDS disease. Practitioners must be cognizant of the economic situation of women involved in prostitution. These women are prostitutes because they are poor and have families to support. Many will continue to engage in high risk activity to continue earning money.

In addressing the knowledge area, prostitutes need accurate information on transmission methods particularly addressing the fear of transmitting the disease to family members. The knowledge on safer sex needs to be improved. Some methods that have been proven successful in other locations include audio visual, anatomically correct models and the very popular "fotonovelas" comic books in Mexico. The foundation for all the educational programs should be based on the language and socioeconomic status of the group (Bracho de Carpio, Carpio-Cedrano, & Anderson, 1990).

There is major need to provide education that would expand the skills of these prostitutes. They need to be better prepared to talk to the clients in order to engage them in using safer sex practices including the use of condoms (de Zalduondo, 1991; Plummer & Ngugi, 1990). The educational process must not be limited to a prostitute's sexual activities with clients, but must include information about sexual activity with husbands and significant others as well. They also need more skills in informing family members and friends about their fears about transmission of the AIDS virus. For those who want to leave this profession, job training skills should be made available (Decker, 1987).

Another important area that should be addressed by practitioners includes the nonjudgmental attitude of the worker which is very important in the development of good working relations with women in this group (Plummer & Ngugi, 1990). The attitudes of the prostitutes must be considered at all times, taking into account the contexts and influence of the culture, including religious beliefs (Bracho de Carpio et al.).

Practitioners should also take into consideration aspects of programs that have been very effective. Outreach programs by health clinics that include prostitutes have worked very well. (Miller, Turner & Moses, 1990).

Practitioners must establish strong working relationships with public health officials on both sides of the border. They must work closely with bar owners, bar managers, and leaders among prostitutes to develop practical approaches for education and protection of the women involved in prostitution in international settings.

Condoms should be made available to prostitutes at no cost in order to enhance the usage. Condoms should be latex with monoxynal-9. Female condoms should be used on a demonstration basis with this group. The ultimate goal is to organize and educate prostitutes to the point that they can accept or reject clients who engage in risky sex.

LIMITATIONS OF THE STUDY

Three basic limitations of this study exist. First, only one population was surveyed, i.e., lower income prostitutes who received health services through a particular clinic. The sample does not reflect prostitutes working in the central district or other areas of Cd. Juarez or American prostitutes in the border city.

Second, in-depth information on the low rates of condom use in general is lacking. Financial, cultural, and religious barriers to the use of condoms, particularly with spouses and significant others, were not fully explored. Furthermore, while fifty-six percent of the prostitutes indicated receiving AIDS information from their clients, the accuracy of such information was not evaluated.

SUGGESTIONS FOR FURTHER RESEARCH

The limitations of this study should be addressed in further research. Broader samples, including prostitutes from both sides of the border, prostitutes working in more affluent areas, prostitutes not receiving health services, and brothels or houses connected to bars should be studied.

A second area for further research is the assessment of the accuracy of information about AIDS received from clients. Little research has been done on this topic, and it would appear that evaluating clients' knowledge could be extremely useful in targeting education efforts.

BIBLIOGRAPHY

Alexander, P. (1988). Response to AIDS: Scapegoating of prostitutes. *Coyote WS Response.*

Bracho de Carpio, A., Carpio-Cedrano, F.F., & Anderson, L. (1990). Hispanic families learning and teaching about AIDS: A participatory approach at the community level. *Hispanic Journal of Behavioral Sciences, 12* (2) 165-176.

Bradbeer, C.S., Thin, R.N., Tan, T., & Thirumoorthy, T. (1988). Prophylaxis against infection in Singaporean prostitutes. *Genitourin Medicine, 64,* 52-53.

Chikwem, J.O., Ola, T.O., Gashau, W., Chikwem, S.D., Bajami, M., & Mambula, S. (1988). Impact of health education on prostitutes' awareness and attitudes to acquired immune deficiency syndrome (AIDS). *Public Health, 102,* 439-445.

Darrow, William W. (1990). Human immunodeficiency virus infection in female prostitutes. In G. de. The (Ed.), *AIDS 89-90* (p.p. 1-17). New York: Medsi/ McGraw-Hill.

Darrow, W.W. et al. (1990). Prostitution, intravenous drug use, and HIV-1 in the United States. In M. Plant (Ed.), *AIDS: Drugs, and prostitution.* London: Routledge, 1990: 18-40.

Dawson, D.A., & Hardy, A.M. (1989). AIDS knowledge and attitudes of Hispanic Americans. *NCHS Advance Data, 166.*

Decker, J.F. (1987). Prostitution as a public health issue. In H. L. Dalton, S. Burris, and the Yale AIDS Project, eds., *AIDS and the law.* New Haven: Yale University Press.

Delacoste, F., & Alexander, P., eds. (1987). *Sex works: writings by women in the sex industry.* San Francisco: Cleis Press.

El Paso City-County Health District (1990). *AIDS Report.*

Goldberg, D.J., Green, S.T., Kingdom, J.C.P. et al. (1988). HIV Infection among female drug-misusing prostitutes in Greater Glasgow. *Communicable Diseases (Scotland), Bulletin 88/12,* 1-3.

Heise, L. (1988). AIDS: New threat to the third world. *World Watch, 1,* 19.

Jaget, C., (Ed.) (1980). *Prostitutes-our life.* Bristol, U.K.: Falling Wall Press.

Johnson, A.M. (1988). Heterosexual transmission of human immune deficiency virus. *British Medical Journal, 296.*

Kreiss, J.K., Koech, D., Plummer, F.A., Holmes, K.K., Lightfoote, M., Piot, P., Ronald, A.R., Ndinya-Achola, J.O., D'Costa, L.J., Roberts, P., Ngugi, E.N., & Quinn, T.C. (1986). AIDS virus infection in Nairobi prostitutes: spread of the epidemic to East Africa. *New England Journal of Medicine, 314* (7), 414-418.

Mann, J.M., Nzilambi, N., Piot, P., Bosenge, N., Kalala, M., Francis, H., Colebunders, R.C., Azila, P.K., Curran, J.W., Quinn, T.C. (1988). HIV infection and associated risk factors in female prostitutes in Kinshasa, Zaire. *Gower Academic Journals Ltd, 0269-9370, 24.*

Miller , H.G., Turner, C.F., & Moses, L.E., (Eds.) (1990). Interventions for female prostitutes. *AIDS: The second decade.* Washington, DC.: National Academy Press.

Pareja, R., Rosario, S., Smith, W., Butler de Lister, M., & Guerrero, E. (1989). Santo Domingo female sex workers' use and handling of condoms: Knowledge and skills. *AIDS Health Promotion Exchange, 2,* 6-9.

Perkins, R., & Bennett, G. (1985). *Being a prostitute: Prostitute women and prostitute men.* Boston, MA.: Allen and Unwin, Inc.

Plant, M.L., Plant, M.A., Peck, D.F., & Setters, J. (1989). The sex industry, alcohol and illicit drugs: Implications for the spread of HIV infection. *British Journal of Addiction, 84,* 53-59.

Plummer, F.A., & Ngugi, E.N. (1990). Prostitutes and their clients in the epidemiology and control of sexually transmitted diseases. (Eds.) *Sexually transmitted diseases.* 2nd Ed. eds. In K.K. Holmes, P. Mardh, P.F. Sparling, & P.J. Wiesner. New York: McGraw-Hill Information Services Company.

Rosenberg, M.J., & Weiner, J.M. (1988). Prostitutes and AIDS: A health department priority? *American Journal of Public Health, 78*(4), 418.

Shaw, S., McChie, J., & Finney, A. (1987). What are poor folk to do? *New Statesman, 113,* 19.

Thomas, R.M., Plant, M.A., Plant, M.L., Sales, D.I. (1989). Risks of AIDS among workers in the "sex industry": Some initial results from a Scottish study. *British Medical Journal, 299,* 148-149.

de Zalduondo, B.O. (1991). Prostitution viewed cross culturally: Toward recontextualizing sex work in AIDS intervention research. *The Journal of Sex Research, 28* (2), 223-248.

Perinatal AIDS:
Permanency Planning
for the African-American Community

Susan Taylor-Brown
Chris Wilczynski
Ellen Moore
Flossie Cohen

SUMMARY. Increasing attention must be given to the psychosocial needs of families with HIV-infected mothers, especially as it relates to permanency planning for children who survive their infected parent(s). Since these families are disproportionately African-American, developing culturally-appropriate services is paramount. Norwood (1988) projected between 52,272 and 72,000 uninfected children will be orphaned in New York City. In Michigan, to understand this problem better, a retrospective chart review utilizing Norwood's model was performed of the families of the 83 infants whose cord blood was positive for maternal HIV antibodies or who were congenitally infected with HIV.

These data have important implications for permanency planning which are presented in the context of their impact on the African-American community. Historically, child welfare has not served African-American children well. A family-centered approach is applied in examining the permanency planning challenges raised.

Susan Taylor-Brown, PhD, MPH, is affiliated with Syracuse University. Chris Wilczynski, MSW, is affiliated with Eastern Michigan University. Ellen Moore, MD, and Flossie Cohen, MD, are affiliated with the Children's Hospital of Michigan and Wayne State University School of Medicine.

Supported by HRSA PHS DHHS BRH PO5032-01-0 and Eastern Michigan University's Spring/Summer Faculty Research Award 1989.

Instrument may be obtained from: Dr. Susan Taylor-Brown, 117 Crescent Hill Road, Pittsford, NY 14534.

INTRODUCTION

The importance of addressing the psychosocial needs of families with Human Immunodeficiency Virus(HIV)-infected mothers is gaining recognition. The care of these families–infected mother/and father, infected child/children, and non-infected children is challenging existing medical and social services. In the rush to provide needed medical care to infected women, permanency planning for the children who survive their infected parent(s) is frequently overlooked.

At this time, AIDS continues to be a stigmatized, terminal illness, especially for women. It threatens an infected woman's ability to connect with others. An infected woman faces the ultimate disconnection from her children–either by her own or her child's death. Jean Baker Miller (1988) explored the impact of disconnections on a woman's relational experience and suggested that emotional dysfunction occurs when women are severed from their primary relationships. Miller and colleagues at the Stone Center developed the relational approach which focuses on reconnecting women to their primary relationships (Fedele & Harrington, 1990). Assisting an HIV-infected woman's ability to reconnect or to remain connected to her children and to plan for them is critical. As Norwood notes, "Since the mothers are usually the last surviving parent, if these HIV-infected women develop Acquired Immunodeficiency Syndrome (AIDS), it is likely that their children will be orphaned" (Norwood, 1988). Families should be assisted in legally formalizing their children's futures. Typically, mothers informally arrange for extended family members or friends to provide for surviving children. Informal custody arrangements are not legally binding and fail to qualify children for necessary services including medical treatment. Norwood estimates that between 52,272 and 72,000 uninfected children will be orphaned in New York City alone. Not only will they be orphaned, many will not have a legal guardian.

Every effort should be made to ensure a stable living arrangement for children whose mothers die. Infected women should be assisted in making permanency plans for their children. Permanency planning should be implemented not only for the infected offspring but for uninfected siblings as well. To develop the necessary supportive services, communities need to systematically understand the impact of HIV-infection on women and children. An accurate assessment of the number of children likely to be orphaned is an important facet of anticipating the need for long-term care. A variety of guardianship options including: extended family placement, long-term foster care, and adoption may be useful in providing for orphaned children.

METHOD

To understand the magnitude of the problem in Michigan, Norwood's model was utilized to calculate the future projections of orphaned children as a result of maternal HIV-infection. A retrospective chart review was conducted using a convenience sample of the 83 children whose cord blood[1] was positive for HIV antibody and were cared for (from June 1985 to April 1989) by the division of Clinical Immunology and the Maternal Infant Center for HIV-infection (MICH). MICH is a tertiary care center providing services to pediatric AIDS patients. The convenience sample was selected from the patient population of MICH which cares for the majority of HIV-infected children in Michigan. Children who were not infected perinatally, e.g., blood transfusion, were excluded from the current study. MICH is unique in that it combines comprehensive care (medical, psychological, and social) for both mothers and children at one site using a case management system.

The children's charts were reviewed using an eighteen item instrument devised by the co-authors to determine the relative numbers of HIV-uninfected and infected children of mothers HIV-infected heterosexually or by IV drug use (IVDU). This data was collected following Norwood's calculations. Norwood (1988) was the first investigator to make projections of the number of infected and uninfected children born to HIV+ women in New York City. Norwood compared the ratio of uninfected offspring to HIV+ offspring by maternal mode of transmission (Heterosexual transmission versus Intravenous transmission). The quantification of HIV disease is an important tool in anticipating families' need and developing needed support services. Next, these figures were compared with Norwood's. Finally, projections were made estimating the number of surviving uninfected and infected offspring for the state of Michigan.

Supplementary demographic data such as age, race/ethnic background, the child's living arrangement at the time of the chart review, and number of siblings was collected to provide more information regarding these children and their families.

The majority of children were born with their cord blood positive for HIV antibody, and a few were older siblings, also perinatally infected. Infants were monitored from birth to ascertain the presence of HIV infection. For the majority of children, it was generally possible to determine HIV infection during the first year of life. For this study, the infants' infection status was categorized into four groups:

1. *Indeterminant*: the infant is generally less than 15 months of age, maternal HIV antibody may still be present, infant is clinically and immunologically well.
2. *Passive Transfer of Maternal Antibody*: infants whose cord blood was positive and who subsequently tested negative, with no other clinical or immunological evidence of infection. These infants are followed for 3 years.
3. *HIV-Infection*: infants with persistently positive HIV antibody as well as other clinical and immunological evidence of HIV infection.
4. *AIDS*: infants with persistent HIV antibody as well as clinical and immunological criteria for AIDS according to Centers for Disease Control (CDC) criteria in January 1989.

RESULTS

Only the 83 infants and positive children (HIV-infected siblings) whose cord blood was HIV antibody positive or presumed to be infected perinatally were included in the present study. Infected adolescents and children infected by blood transfusions were excluded.

During the perinatal period, infants will test HIV+ reflecting the presence of maternal HIV antibodies. During the first eighteen months of life, in the majority of cases, it is possible to determine whether the infant is infected or merely had his/her mother's HIV antibodies present at birth (passive transfer). For a small number of patients, their HIV status is not clearly discernible and they are classified indeterminant. Indeterminant cases are followed regularly until diagnosis is confirmed.

Of the 83 children, 19 (23%) were HIV infected, 10 (12%) had AIDS, 27 (32.5%) had passive transfer of maternal HIV-antibody and 27(32.5%) indeterminant, representing an infection rate of 52% (Table I).[2]

The majority of the 83 children (70%) were less than two years of age. Three infants (4%) were deceased. The male to female distribution was almost equal (47% and 53%, respectively), and the majority were African-American (88%) (Table II).

These 83 children belonged to 71 families and most (77%) were being cared for by their parents or relatives, while 15 (18%) were in foster care. Eleven (15%) of the families had more than one child whose cord blood was positive for HIV antibody. Ten families had two children whose cord blood was positive and one family

TABLE I: HIV status of infants and children whose cord blood was positive for HIV-antibody by year of referral

YEAR	HIV-INFECTED	AIDS*	PASSIVE TRANSFER	INDETERMINANT+	TOTAL
1985	0	2	2	0	4
1986	3	2	9	0	14
1987	6	3	15	4	28
1988	9	3	1	11	24
1989(Jan-Mar)	1	0	0	12	13
TOTAL	19	10	27	27	83

*CDC DEFINITION
+ NOT CLEAR WHETHER HIV-INFECTED, FEW LOST TO FOLLOW-UP

TABLE II: Socio-demographic Information
Number (Percentage)
%

AGE		
≤1 YEAR	32	(39)
>1 YR. ≤ 2	26	(31)
>2 YRS. ≤ 3	14	(17)
>3 YRS. ≤ 4	3	(3)
>4 YRS. ≤ 5	4	(5)
OVER 5 YRS.	1	(1)
DECEASED	3	(4)
	83	(100)
SEX		
MALE	39	(47)
FEMALE	44	(53)
	83	(100)
RACE/ETHNIC BACKGROUND		
AFRICAN-AMERICAN	73	(88)
WHITE	10	(12)
	83	(100)
LIVING SITUATION AT THE TIME OF THE STUDY		
IN-HOME	44	(53)
OTHER RELATIVE	20	(24)
FOSTER CARE	15	(18)
ADOPTED	1	(1)
DECEASED	3	(4)
	83	(100)

had 3 children. In addition to the 83 children, there were 136 additional siblings whose ages ranged from 1 year to 26 years, with an average of 3.21 children per family.

Since this is a study of perinatal transmission of HIV, all of the mothers were infected. Of the 71 mothers, 14 (20%) were suspected to have been infected heterosexually, 57 (80%) were suspected to have been infected by IV drug use. None had AIDS at the time of delivery, three developed AIDS at 5 months, 9 months, and 18 months after delivery.

Application of Norwood's Model

Norwood compared the relative numbers of uninfected to infected children among a group of heterosexually-infected and a second group who contracted HIV-infection from drug use. Next she calculated projections for the number of surviving uninfected children. In the present study, projections of surviving infected offspring for the state of Michigan are provided.

In Michigan, women infected heterosexually on average, have 2.75 times the number of non-HIV-infected children as they have HIV-infected children; women infected by drug use on average have 6.71 times the number of non-HIV-infected to every infected child. These findings are in reverse of those reported by Norwood (Table III). She found that women infected heterosexually had 7.3 times the number of non-HIV-infected to HIV-infected children and women infected by IV-drug use had 3 times the number of non-HIV-infected to HIV-infected children.

Projection of Infected and Uninfected Offspring in Michigan

Projections of the number of infected and uninfected offspring are presented in this paper and should help providers anticipate future planning needs.

From July-December 1988, the Michigan Department of Health, in collaboration with the Centers for Disease Control, carried out a needle-stick investigation of all live births in the state. This entailed anonymously testing the cord blood of infants born in the state. The preliminary results indicate that for every 10,000 births, 6 children were antibody positive. In the 6 county area surrounding Detroit the rate was 11/10,000 and the remainder of the state was 2/10,000. Based upon these figures there are estimated to be 1,300-

TABLE III: Norwood's assessment of uninfected and infected children and Taylor-Brown et al.'s replication

	TOTAL MOTHERS	NON-HIV CHILDREN	TOTAL HIV+	NON-HIV RATIO TO HIV+	AVERAGE NON-HIV
NORWOOD'S STUDY HETERO-SEXUALLY INFECTED	3 0	59	8	7.3:1	1.97
IV DRUG INFECTED	3 4	71	23	3:1	2.08
TAYLOR-BROWN *et al.* HETEROSEXUALLY INFECTED*	1 4	22	8	2.75:1	1.57
IV DRUG INFECTED*√	5 7	141	21	6.71:1	2.66

[*N=4 Missing Cases; √=27 children with indeterminant status excluded from this analysis, since HIV status is undetermined at this time (23 children (IVDU)=indeterminant, 4 children (hetero)=indeterminant)]

1,400 HIV-infected women of childbearing age (15-45 yrs.) in Michigan (Personal Communication with Bill Hall, Ph.D., of the Michigan Department of Public Health, Data Surveillance Section on June 26, 1989). If 80% of these women develop AIDS or related lethal diseases, that leaves a low estimate of 1,040 mothers with HIV-associated mortality and a high of 1,120 mothers with HIV-associated mortality.

Given the overall average of 2.7 non-HIV-infected children per mother, it is projected these women would leave behind between 2,208 to 3,024 non-HIV-infected offspring. Our results indicate an average (HIV-infected + AIDS/Total # of mothers) of .60 HIV-infected children per infected mother of childbearing age. This figure includes women who had multiple antibody positive cord blood children. This results in a projection of 624 to 672 infected children needing specialized services. Some of these infected children will precede their mothers in death.

DISCUSSION

This study is an effort to quantify the magnitude of perinatal AIDS in Michigan in order to facilitate long-term permanency planning for infected and uninfected children of HIV-infected women. These data are preliminary and may not be applicable to other geographical areas. For example, when compared to national data, the sample disproportionately represents African-Americans, does not include Hispanics and the mode of transmission was disproportionately the result of IV drug use.

The reversal of ratios for women in New York and Detroit suggests that the mode of transmission classification may be unreliable. How does one know, for instance, how a drug-addicted woman, who had multiple sexual partners became infected? If only 5 to 6% of the women are mistaken, the figures would be quite different. It follows that, to achieve accurate results, the samples should be much larger and great care should be exercised in the questioning of patients to determine the mode of transmission or it may be more reliably based on behavioral lifestyle.

Too often children perinatally infected with HIV are viewed in isolation, ignoring their families and their needs. As McGonigel (1989) reports, "one commonly held view is that most children with AIDS do not even have families." Both Norwood's and our study document that infected children do have families and that these families are confronting terminal illness in two or more of their family members. For the HIV-infected mothers, the importance of maintaining their bonds with their children deserves particular emphasis. The women and their families will need support services if this is to happen.

As previously noted, AIDS continues to be a fatal illness and the majority of these children will be orphaned during the next decade. The challenge of pediatric AIDS is developing a mosaic of services which help families function while confronting life-threatening illness. The remainder of this article applies a family-centered approach to the permanency planning challenges. Since the majority of infected children both nationally and in our sample are African-American, these findings are discussed in the context of their relevance to the African-American community. The national response to pediatric AIDS must incorporate the African-American community in all phases of service delivery. This will help to ensure that children receive ethnically-appropriate service which foster family preservation and competence. The African-American community has a rich history of responding compassionately and adaptively to adversity. The magnitude of this problem mandates that the total society mount a response. It is too grave a burden for any one community to bear.

Coping with Multiple Losses

With the perinatally HIV-infected child serving as the index for a family confronting HIV-infection in multiple family members, the data powerfully depicts the devastating impact of perinatal AIDS on affected families. Not only are the needs of those infected paramount, but equal attention must be given to the family members who are uninfected. The uninfected members are dealing with the disease progression and deaths of two or more loved ones.

One of the most painful realities is that HIV+ family members frequently do not disclose the diagnosis to family members because of the stigma. This results in illness and death surrounded by secrecy and dealt with indirectly. Family members know that something serious is happening but may be totally unaware of the diagnosis and its life-threatening nature. This secrecy compounds the trauma of coping with life-threatening illness. Many families bury their loved ones surrounded by shame and secrecy. Further, many of the children are young and their ability to cope with the multiple losses is limited. This creates painful realities for providers and families alike.

While it may be impossible to conquer AIDS related death, it is possible to work with a family facing multiple losses. First, medical care providers are often the only people aware of the diagnosis. As a result, the medical team has an opportunity to help the family anticipate and cope with the inherent losses by offering a setting to explore these toxic issues. Psychosocial services can be offered to HIV-affected families. Helping HIV-infected family members develop videotapes for surviving members is one example of innovative approaches to coping with impending loss. These tapes create an opportunity for family members to share their story, tell their family that they love them, and to provide guidance for the future (Wiener, 1990 and Taylor-Brown, in press). If videotapes are not possible, letters or audiotapes can help family members cope with the loss. While the professional cannot totally remove the pain associated with these losses, s/he can buffer the consequences.

Another component of providing care to HIV-affected families is the development of a continuum of services which facilitate the family's ability to stay together.

Support Services: The Need
for Ongoing Intermittent Care of Children

HIV disease episodically incapacitates those who are infected. With improved survival rates, the illness is approaching a chronic disease model for those receiving adequate medical care. During illness episodes of either the mother or child(ren), care for the other children is an important facet of care. At times, the mother may be unable to care for her children. Babysitting, respite care or temporary out of home care may be needed. When a family is unable to arrange this care, alternatives will be needed.

While the AIDS epidemic may be stressing our current resources to capacity, it may also be creating a unique opportunity for growth and consolidation of child welfare services into a model that truly fosters family preservation with outside resources being brought in to support and supplement families as needed. Communities need to gain a greater awareness of the incidence and prevalence of perinatal HIV-infection to assist the child welfare system in responding to this situation in a thoughtful, proactive rather than crisis-oriented, reactive fashion. For Michigan, the data suggest that women infected by IV-drug use have more children on average than those infected heterosexually. This group of women should be targeted for intensive services to preserve the family for as long as possible and to facilitate permanency planning for surviving children.

Dr. G. Woodruff (1989) defined family-centered care as "Families defining who they are and what services they need." Family-centered care is a philosophy of practice in which families and health care providers form a partnership to care for children with handicapping conditions. Typically these services are community based. Families are trained to provide support to others facing similar situations. This model seems particularly applicable to pediatric AIDS. The Association for Care of Children's Health hosted the first family meeting on Pediatric AIDS which addressed the application of a family-centered approach to care for HIV-infected children. Natural mothers, grandmothers, aunts, and foster mothers, foster fathers and adoptive mothers all participated in the meeting. At the meeting, McGonigel (1989) distinguished between "given" and "chosen" families. For the natural, foster, or adoptive family, "given" refers to biologically related family members who may or may not accept the HIV-infected child. The stigma of AIDS has resulted in rejection of the children in some of these families. As a result, families have sought out new "chosen" family members to assume the roles of the absent relatives. A "chosen" family may include the natural mother and foster care family working together to care for the child.

A family-centered approach to permanency planning mandates that the family's needs be taken into account. First and foremost, mothers should be supported in developing long-term plans for their children. Early assessment and intervention with these families may help to lessen the emotional stress(es) of losing a parent and/or children. A long-term care plan should be devised for each child within the family. Clearly, the timing of interventions is important. A woman grappling with the implications of her own diagnosis may not be ready for the finality of permanency planning. In order to make permanence plans, a woman must acknowledge her own terminal illness coupled with the realization that her child is infected as a result of her infection. While the majority of women do not know they are HIV-infected until the baby's cord blood tests positive for HIV-antibody, they still must deal with the pain and guilt of transmitting the illness to their offspring. It is imperative to balance hope for the future with the somewhat paradoxical reality of permanency planning.

The child's extended family may be an important resource for infected children. Boyd-Franklin (1989) emphasizes the importance of the extended family in understanding the lives of many African-

American families. She calls for an expansion of the field of our vision of African-American families from a focus on the nuclear family model to the incorporation of an extended family and multi-systems model (p. 42). Boyd-Franklin (1989, p. 43) notes that:

> For many African-American extended families, reciprocity–or the process of helping each other and exchanging and sharing support as well as goods and services–is a very central part of their lives.

Extended families may include blood relatives and non-related friends. Inclusion of extended family members in long-term planning may help the mothers and children remain together. It may also comfort the mother to have a trusted family member or friend caring for her children. When the mother is too ill to care for her children, episodic temporary care may be needed and permanent placement may be needed ultimately. Consideration should be given to ensuring the stability of extended familial relationships for the infected and uninfected children. Efforts should be made to provide continuity of care in order to minimize the child's losses and to reinforce his/her attachments to primary care givers. At times, both mother and child may need residential care. Simon House in Detroit is developing a group living situation for women and children.

Family Preservations

Public Law 96-272, the Child Welfare Reform and Adoption Assistance Act of 1980 mandates the development of services to prevent the placement of children outside of their own homes. Maternal HIV infection poses unique challenges to child welfare's ability to preserve families. There hasn't been a comparable illness, devastating to the family, and resulting in repeated maternal incapacity and death. Maternal illness can be difficult to predict which creates service delivery challenges. Although the child welfare system is mandated to preserve the family, the system is not experienced in responding to the need for immediate and sometimes repeated intermittent care. As the mother's illness progresses, it is likely that she will be hospitalized, creating a need for intermittent care, and the family may need extensive support in order to stay together. The Report of the Child Welfare League of America's Task Force on Children with HIV Infection (1988, p. 25) strongly supported family preservation by recommending:

> The preservation of the family unit, whether biological, foster, adoptive or extended family should be a primary consideration when dealing with HIV-infected children/clients to the extent possible. Treatment of the family as a unit is critical to the prevention and treatment of the disease and should be recognized as such.

With the family unit as the focal system, social workers can work with community agencies to provide the necessary services.

Historically, African-American children have not been well served by the child welfare system. Billingsley and Giovannoni (1972) traced the unresponsiveness of child welfare to the needs of African-American children. As a result, informal adoptions developed separate from the child welfare system. Informal adoption in the African-American community has a rich history which Hill (1977) described as an informal social service network that has been an integral part of the African-American community since the days of slavery. Informal adoption is the process of relatives or friends caring for minor children whose parents are unable to care for them. A family-centered approach to the provision of services suggests that efforts be made to enlist family members or close friends in the care of the surviving children. Legal guardianship determines who is able to obtain the needed services for the child. For example, unless a grandmother was designated the guardian while caring for her grandchild, she would not be eligible to obtain health care insurance or other benefits. Incorporation of informal adoption arrangements should be an integral component in caring for those affected by perinatal AIDS. To accomplish this, efforts must be made to have informal adoptions recognized legally, allowing children to receive necessary services. Some social service agencies have policies restricting the use of extended family members for foster care (Born Hooked, 1989; Invisible Emergency, 1987). Trupin called for changes in the system to recognize and support grandparents (Born Hooked, 1989). Further, some agencies require extended family members to file neglect petitions in order to receive services. To ask a family member to file a neglect petition against a relative would add further stress to the family. McGonigel (1989) reported that support and resources available to natural parents and other caregiving members of a child's biological family varied from those available to foster parents. Biological families need supportive services if they are to continue to care for their infected family members. All caregivers should have equal access to needed services. All of these policies should be reviewed in light of the situations created by this illness.

In some instances, it may be that the children are best served outside of the home but every effort should be made to maintain the primary familial relationships. Dr. V. Anderson (With Loving Arms, 1989) notes that for children, separation from a parent is more painful and understandable to the child than the child's own impending death; that is, the child may comprehend the experience of parental death more directly than his/her own impending loss. Thus, even if a mother is unable to care directly for her child, she should be assisted in maintaining a meaningful relationship with her children. As noted earlier, children may need repeated out-of-home care as a result of the mother's illness. Children will benefit from having as much caretaker continuity as is possible. Parents and foster care parents may work together as the child's chosen family.

When kinship care is not possible, other alternatives include foster care, adoption, and group care. Children should be placed in the least restrictive environment available (Anderson, 1986). The African-American community should be the primary resource in these efforts.

A number of innovative programs have been initiated around the country (Gurdin, 1989; McCarley, 1989; and West, 1989). Efforts to recruit foster care and adoptive families have been successful (Ettinger, 1988; Gurdin, 1989; Gurdin & Anderson, 1987). Extensive training of staff and foster care parents, enhanced reimbursement, and ongoing support of foster care parents are central to these programs. Foster care or adoptive parents have the right to know the child's serostatus (Anderson, 1986; Boland, 1987) and equally need to protect the child's privacy. A child's serostatus should be confidential and shared only when necessary for the child's care. Deception by the child welfare agency and social work staff can create serious problems in the relationships with current and prospective foster parents (Lockhart & Wodarski, 1989).

Adoption of HIV-infected children offers them the stability of a permanent home and, unlike foster care, allows the parents to direct the child's treatment. A major obstacle to adoption is the medical costs associated with caring for a pediatric AIDS patient. Tourse and Gunderson (1988) note that adoptive parents are financially responsible for medical costs and suggest that subsidies be considered to encourage adoption; or perhaps these families will be restricted to providing long-term foster care in order to preserve the child's medical coverage.

Children already within the child welfare system may be at-risk for HIV infection as a result of past exposure to high-risk events including sexual abuse, sexual activity or IVDU. These children need careful and ongoing psychosocial and medical monitoring. Current drug therapies confirm that HIV infection, while not curable, is definitely treatable, improving and decreasing morbidity, making early diagnosis an important goal. While universal testing doesn't seem prudent, testing should be based on exposure to at-risk behaviors and relevant medical indications. Children entering foster care should be given medical evaluations which include evaluation of at-risk behaviors. Drug exposure of infants is a contributing factor lending to out-of-home placement. For example, in California, Halfon reports that up to 60% of drug-exposed infants have been placed in foster care (Born Hooked, 1989). Frequently, these infants are medically cleared for discharge from the hospital but are unable to leave because their families are unable to care for them and alternative placements are not available (Hegarty et al., 1988). These infants are referred to as boarder babies. This problem is compounded by the fact that these children are at increased risk for HIV infection. Hegarty et al. (1988) calculated the average lifetime cost for an HIV-infected child as $90,347 per child with boarder babies having a mean length of stay nearly four times longer than those with homes (339 days versus 89 days). Rice (Born Hooked, 1989) reported that Washington, DC had 41 children classified as "boarder babies." Not only are boarder babies expensive, but a hospital is not the least restrictive environment for the child. For infants with maternal antibodies determined present at birth, ongoing medical surveillance will establish whether the infant is infected or not. Their siblings should be monitored for infection also.

Foster care parents can play an important role in care of these children. Education of foster care parents may facilitate early identification of infected children and encourage retention of those children in their current foster care placement.

PREVENTION

The need for prevention is apparent. Efforts must be directed toward stopping the spread of HIV in our communities. Too many women are unaware that they are infected and are at-risk for transmitting the illness. The majority of these women are in their childbearing years. The reported 52% infection rate of children perinatally infected makes prevention imperative. Women need education regarding the risks involved in future pregnancies so that they can make informed choices. Approximately ninety percent of the women in the current study found out they were HIV+ following the child's birth, suggesting that intensive educational efforts should be targeted to women prior to pregnancy. Women entering their child-bearing years or those of child-bearing age who are not currently infected consist of another important target group. In Washington, D.C., there is an innovative effort targeted to the 13 to 17 year old group, who will be trained to do AIDS education among their peers (Hill, 1989).

Perinatal AIDS poses a serious challenge to our communities, particularly the African-American community. Members of two generations are being lost. The impact of this loss will be increasingly felt as the incidence of HIV infection and its associated mortality progresses. Extensive community outreach and involvement is necessary to respond to the need for nonparental care.

Efforts targeted to the African-American churches and community based agencies currently serving the African-American community should be helpful in recruiting foster care parents. The Southern

Christian Leadership Conference/Women's Organizational Movement for Equality Now (SCLC/WOMEN) organized a conference, AIDS and the African-American Community, which explored why African-Americans and other minorities may not be receiving or adopting adequate health care information from mainstream health care systems. A community handbook was developed, presenting practical approaches to decrease the risk of HIV infection. Both SCLC/WOMEN (1987) and Streat (1987) cite issues indigenous to the African-American community that may impede education of at-risk individuals including the widespread belief that AIDS is a gay white male's disease. To date, the church leaders have generally not been supportive. As the epidemic progresses, community leaders, particularly from the church, need to be utilized in developing AIDS programs and overcoming some of the current barriers to successful AIDS prevention. Biological, foster and adoptive families can benefit from emotional support, transportation, respite care, and other supportive community services. SCLC/ WOMEN and other community groups are assuming a leadership role in combating the stigma of AIDS. But it is the responsibility of all America to care for these children; no one segment of society can be expected to carry the responsibility of the epidemic. As Dr. Reed Tuckson (1989) eloquently states: "Our society will be judged by how it responded to or failed to respond to the AIDS epidemic."

In addition to AIDS' training, workers will need to develop an in-depth understanding of the skills used in the assessment of extended family networks, to obtain necessary and limited resources, to assist the family to cope with multiple deaths, to plan placement of children whose HIV status is uncertain, and to cope with the personal stress associated with working with a terminally-ill and stigmatized patient group. An integral component of training should address the development of cultural competence by workers providing services to infected women and children, who are disproportionately people of color. Gray and Nybell (1990) make four assumptions about services to African-American children: (1) that child welfare service takes place in a cultural context; (2) that African-American families require a culturally relative non-deficit perspective on African-American culture; (3) that service providers acquire an analytical approach to culture and factual knowledge about the cultural behavior of clients; and, (4) that the staff be prepared, through training, to implement a cultural knowledge base in transactions with African-American families and must have the supervisory and policy supports.

Finally, research evaluating the development of permanency plans for infected children and their uninfected siblings should lead to a more responsive and appropriate care system for these children and their families.

NOTES

1. The blood contained in an infant's umbilical cord is tested which is indicative of exposure to HIV. The umbilical cord is tested for indication of exposure to HIV.

2. The infection rate was calculated by: Infection rate = (HIV-infected + AIDS)/(HIV-infected + AIDS + Passive Transfer). The children whose HIV-status was indeterminant were excluded from this calculation since their HIV-status was not definitive at the time of the study.

REFERENCES

Anderson, G. (1986). *Children and AIDS: The challenge for child welfare.* Washington, D.C.: Child Welfare Press.

Billingsley, A. & Giovannoni, J. (1970). *Children of the storm: Black children and American child welfare.* NY: Harcourt Brace Jovanovich.

Boland, M. (1989, April 6). *View from the front line.* Paper presented at AIDS: Infants and Children Conference, Forum for Health Care Planning, Washington, D.C.

Boland, M., Tasker, A., Evans, P. & Kereszlez, J. (1987). *Helping children with AIDS: The role of the child welfare worker. Public Welfare, 45*(1), 23-80.

Born hooked: Confronting the impact of perinatal substance abuse. Select Committee on Children, Youth and Families. Washington, D.C.: U.S. House of Representatives (1989, April 27).

Boyd-Franklin, N. (1989). *Black families in therapy: A multisystems approach.* NY: Guilford Press.

Doubleday, W. (1987). *Death, dying and AIDS.* In V. Gong & N. Rudick (eds.), *AIDS: Facts and issues* (pp. 291-302). New Brunswick: Rutgers University Press.

Ettinger, P. (1988). *Children with HIV infection and their families: An assessment and recommendations.* A Report to the Philadelphia Commission on AIDS. Available from Leonard Davis Institute of Health Economics, University of Pennsylvania, 3641 Locust Walk, Philadelphia, PA 19104.

Gray, S. & Nybell, L. (1990, Nov.). Issues in black family preservation. *Child Welfare, LXIX*(6), 513-524.

Gurdin, P. (1989, April 6). *Housing and foster care.* Paper presented at AIDS: Infants and Children Conference, Forum for Health Care Planning, Washington, D.C.

Gurdin, P. & Anderson, C. (1987). Quality care for children: AIDS specialized foster family homes. *Child Welfare, LXV*(4), 291-302.

Hegarty, J., Abrams, E., Hutchingson, V., Nicholas, S., Suarez, M. & Hegarty, M. (1988, October 7). The medical care costs of Human Immunodeficiency Virus-infected children in Harlem. *JAMA, 260* (13), 1901-5.

Hill, A. (1989, January). Coping with HIV positive children. *Social Work Today, 20*(19), 13-15.

Hill, R. (1977). *Informal adoption among Black families.* Washington, DC: Urban League.

Invisible emergency: Children and AIDS in New York. Available from Citizens Committee for Children, 105 E. 22nd St., NY, NY 10010, 1987.

Lockhart, L. & Wodarski, J. (1989, May). Facing the unknown: Children and Adolescents with AIDS. *Social Work,* 215-221.

McCarley, J. (1989, April 6). *Supporting children and their families.* Paper presented at AIDS: Infants and Children Conference, Forum for Health Care Planning, Washington, DC.

McGonigel, M. (1989). *Family meeting on pediatric AIDS.* Washington, DC: ACCH.

Miller, J. (1988). *Connection, disconnections, and violations. Work in Progress, 33.* Wellesley, MA; Stone Center Working Paper Series.

Norwood, C. (1988). *AIDS orphans in New York City: Projected numbers and policy demands.* Washington, DC: National Women's Health Network Report.

Norwood, C. (1988, July). Alarming rise in deaths. *Ms,* 65-67.

Oleske, J. (1989, April 6). *View from the front line.* Paper presented at AIDS: Infants and Children Conference, Forum for Health Care Planning, Washington, DC.

Southern Christian Leadership Conference (1987). *AIDS in the Black community.* Paper presented at the SCLC/WOMEN Conference, Atlanta, GA: SCLC.

Report of the Child Welfare League of America task force on AIDS and HIV infection (1988). Washington, D.C.: Child Welfare League of America.

Streat, T. (1987). *AIDS prevention in the Black community.* In M. Helquist (Ed.). *Working with AIDS* (p. 142-45). San Francisco, CA: University of San Francisco Press.

Surgeon General's Report (1987). *Children with special health care needs. DHHS Publication,* No. 184-020/65654 HRS/D/MC 87-2.

Task Force on Pediatric AIDS (1988). Pediatric guidelines for infection control of Human Immunodeficiency Virus in hospitals, medical offices, schools, and other settings. *Pediatrics 82*(5), 801-7.

Task Force on Pediatric AIDS (1988). Perinatal Human Immunodeficiency Virus infection. *Pediatrics, 82*(6), 941-44.

Taylor-Brown, S. (In press). HIV+ women: Finding a voice in the AIDS pandemic. In V. Lynch, G. Lloyd, & M. Fimbres (eds). *The expanding face of AIDS.* Westport, Conn.: Greenwood Pub.

The hidden risk among adolescents: Program at Montefiore Medical Center. Children with AIDS, 1(7), 1-4, (1989).

Tourse, P. & Gundersen, L. (1988, May-June). Adopting and fostering children with AIDS: Policies in Progress. *Children Today,* 4-7.

Tuckson, R. (1989, April 6). *View from the front line.* Paper presented at AIDS: Infants and Children Conference, Forum for Health Care Planning, Washington, DC.

West, P. (1989, May 23). *The AIDS crisis: Impact on program and policy.* Paper presented at Midwest Regional Training Conference, Child Welfare League of America.

Wiener, L. & Septimus, A. (1991). Psychosocial consideration and support for the child and family. In P. Pizzo (ed.) *Pediatric AIDS* (pp. 577-594).

With loving arms. Videotape available from Child Welfare Association. Washington, DC: Child Welfare League of America, 1989.

Women ignored in research on AIDS (1988, Oct/Nov/Dec) *National NOW Times,* 6.

Woodruff, G. (1989, April 6). *Coordinating community resources.* Paper presented at AIDS: Infants and Children Conference, Forum for Health Care Planning, Washington, DC.

Woodruff, G. & Sterzin, E. (1988, May-June). The transagency approach: A model for serving children with HIV infection and their families. *Children Today,* 9-14.

AIDS:
Health Care Intervention Models
for Communities of Color

Victor De La Cancela
Audrey McDowell

SUMMARY. Health Care approaches to AIDS interventions for individuals of color must include multi-cultural competence and community health center involvement. Equally important is the formulation of policy initiatives that translate into an empowering human services delivery system. This article suggests corresponding strategies that directly relate to people of color.

INTRODUCTION

The HIV/AIDS pandemic has exposed the inadequacies of the U.S. health and hospital care system in a dramatic manner. Specifically, it has shown the system's failure to provide universal access to culturally competent and language appropriate treatment and disease prevention. Concomitantly it has revealed the shortsightedness of developing large acute care hospital facilities at the expense of neighborhood level comprehensive health centers. As such, AIDS has highlighted the need for community-based service delivery, progressive social policy, and strategies for empowerment in research, treatment, and prevention targeted to persons of color.

This article discusses community health care intervention models that address AIDS in communities of color at both the service de-

Victor De La Cancela, PhD, is Senior Vice President for Primary Care Development and Audrey McDowell, MA, is an Intern (Urban Policy) at New York City Health and Hospitals Corporation, 125 Worth Street, New York, NY 10013.

livery and policy levels. It presents the premise that health care workers must "respect" people of color before they can effectively intervene against AIDS in communities of color. Next, it presents the argument that because people of color need a comprehensive, culturally competent approach to AIDS within a biopsychosocial context that is often not available in an acute care hospital, a more likely setting for the delivery of ongoing AIDS care is the community based health center. Finally, it recommends interventions and policies that can enable health care institutions to better serve people of color.

PEOPLE OF COLOR:
SIMILARITIES VS. DIFFERENCES

We define "people of color" as those who have ethnic roots and cultural heritages in Africa, the Caribbean, Asia and the Pacific Islands, and the indigenous people of North, South and Central America. These are people with a triple health care legacy that includes folk healers, "colonial" medical interventions and modern western medicine (McCartney, 1988). However, it is important to state that although these groups share somewhat similar U. S. histories of racial oppression and cultural imperialism, they are not easily lumped together as this creates the danger that one generic approach might be assumed feasible for intervention in all ethnic communities (Campos, 1988). Additionally, there is the hazard that similar to stereotyping, aggregating diverse people into an amorphous "minority" grouping can magnify alleged cultural attributes while concrete social, cultural and economic realities are ignored (Rendon, 1984).

Acknowledging that a tension exists between overemphasizing either people of color's differences and similarities or their within group differences, it is still useful to discuss some groups together since most people of color in the United States experience a "mainstream" approach to health care that does not fully meet their needs because of its Eurocentric focus. Given the structural similarity of the socioeconomic situation that faces various groups of color, many of the necessary interventions will often be conceptually similar, but the specifics of implementation may vary.

There are several differences in communities of color that are particularly important in AIDS related work. First, the incidence of AIDS varies by group. For example, Menedez et al. (1990) report that in New York City Puerto Ricans represent the group most severely affected by AIDS, with cumulative age-adjusted mortality among males significantly higher than among African-Americans, Caucasians or other Latino males. Nationally, cumulative AIDS incidence reports by birthplace indicate that Puerto Ricans are the most disproportionately affected by AIDS (Selik et al., 1989).

The amount of knowledge about AIDS incidence in different communities of color also varies. For example, there are reports that the rate of HIV infection (HIV+) is currently unknown in Indian/Native American communities and that insensitive attempts by the Indian Health Service or Centers for Disease Control to determine prevalence will be resisted as yet another Anglo dominated bureaucratic intrusion (Tafoya, 1991). People of color have generally been excluded from HIV research for a number of reasons, including: the stereotyped view that Latinos, African-Americans and IVDUs are unreliable in keeping appointments or for follow-up (Holmberg, 1988); the assumption that IV drug use skews data due to presence of drugs in the body (Kolata, 1991); and lack of provisions for transportation to research sites and onsite child care for participants. Some people of color exclude themselves because they are hostile towards the "white research" system which "experiments" on them for the sake of careers (Kolata, 1991).

A related issue is the fact that various ethnic/racial groups have differing levels of representation in AIDS research. Recently, there have been yearly increases in the percentage of African-American women participants in clinical trials. On the contrary, Latina representation in these trials has peaked and plateaued (Cotton, Feinberg & Finkelstein, 1991). This is important because inadequate representation of women of color in trials perpetuates a system of drug research and development that is based primarily on Caucasian males' biopsychosocial characteristics.

Communities of color affected by AIDS may also view hospitals and other health care institutions differently. For example, African-

American patients may be fearful and resentful of care provided by trainees and "prejudiced" health professionals. Latinos sometimes view hospitals as a last resort used only for emergencies (Petrovich, 1987) or a place to die in and thus resist admission. Native Americans value children highly and therefore have difficulty with hospital policies that restrict children from being visitors.

Persons of color may also have differing cultural approaches to illness and the healing process. For both Latinos and Native Americans, family contacts and networks are extremely important, but Indian society requires agreement so strongly that major medical decisions might await input from distant family or community members before providers are allowed to act (McKusick, 1991b). Traditional healers are not only important in such consultation, they have, as have Native educators and counselors, proven to be quick to respond to people with AIDS (PWAs) and to integrate spiritual teachings, values and rituals with western treatment, e.g., sweat lodge ceremonies, vision quests, drumming groups, tribal gatherings and experiences in the woods (Rowell, 1990). Other examples are Asians and Pacific Islanders who view discussing illness or death as a self-fulfilling prophecy, and groups like the Hmong who do not use written languages. A final thought to bear in mind regarding differences and similarities among people of color is that AIDS education messages must be designed for those who have assimilated into the dominant culture as well as those who have not (Salas Rojas, 1992).

RESPECTING PEOPLE OF COLOR

In reaching out to visible racial/ethnic groups, health care workers may find that some will a priori suspect the sincerity of AIDS workers' concern about their health status. This response is not unreasonable especially since the European American scientific community has been guilty of making racist "findings," for example, that Africans are equivalent to lobotomized Europeans or that Puerto Ricans suffer uniquely from hysteria-schizophrenia (Rendon, 1984). The most heinous racist study that African-Americans recall in this vein is the 40 year Tuskegee experiment from 1932 to 1972 conducted by the Public Health Service to determine the effects of untreated syphilis on African-American males who were poor and illiterate (Broyles, 1991).

Given this background, health care workers need to explicitly show "respect" for people of color before they can address their AIDS concerns. Educational models must stem from this basis of respect, because it would be impossible to succeed in AIDS work with persons of color without respecting who they are and what they believe. As one health worker reports, you have to "devote time and energy" to addressing the concerns of persons affected by AIDS (PAA) because a dismissal out of hand "turns off" the listener to further intervention (De Parle, 1990). A necessary component of this respect is identifying and utilizing the labels by which a particular community refers to itself. Hence, it is not merely an issue of semantics whether one speaks of Hispanics, Blacks, Orientals and Indians or Latinos, African, Asian and Native Americans; rather it is reflective of how a particular group liberates itself from the labels applied to them by others. As Helms (1990) has clearly stated, the appellation issue is one of empowerment since a people are less powerful when their "identity is defined by outgroup members and it is indistinguishable from other disempowered groups."

Respect is also evident in acknowledging world views and priority agendas of people of color. For example, knowledge of the socio-politically influenced time perspectives and shorter lifespans of Latinos and African Americans would suggest that prevention messages should focus on the "here and now," not some distant future which they may never reach (Rosenthal, 1990). Likewise, AIDS media campaigns should be tied to the issues that oppressed communities and their leaders care about and work on, such as drug prevention, the future of children, violence and crime reduction.

Lee and Fong (1990) claim that Asian and Pacific Islander communities have not benefitted from the application of Caucasian gay oriented safer sex models nor from approaches that were found to be effective for Latinos and African-Americans. Their report suggests, in conclusion, that health care workers must respect each patient's cultural individuality, instead of assuming that interventions that have worked in other situations will be appropriate for every patient.

BIOPSYCHOSOCIAL APPROACHES ARE REQUIRED

In keeping with the concept of respect, the biological syndrome of AIDS must be approached psychosocially so that targeted persons of color are not alienated or made to feel expendable. Some people have social histories of being unwanted and of discrimination even before AIDS due to their drug use or sexual practices, while others feel this way as a result of bias manifested against them on racial grounds. If they become HIV+ their social realities may include: rejection by their religious networks; or lack of access to medical care due to poor housing, finances, insurance, distance from service settings, or language differences (Cohen & Weisman, 1986). In addition, their caregiver networks may also be overwhelmed by the lack of adequate resources or have members suffering from AIDS themselves (Cohen, Weisman & Vazquez, 1988).

There are of course additional losses caused by the stigma attached to AIDS. For example, women of color may avoid seeking treatment for fear that their children will be removed from them or excluded from schools (Cowley, Hager & Marshall, 1990). This fear may be especially pronounced for women who have histories of IV drug use. In many states such use may expose them to legal charges of child neglect or abuse. Indeed within certain circles there has been talk of defining women who are HIV+ and pregnant as "prenatal child abusers." These realities engender multiple stressors for persons of color affected by AIDS. When grown children and their families must move back into the homes of their parents additional stress is created. Travel across state and national borders to return to families of origin and birthplaces indicates that crisis intervention, family and even network therapy might be necessary (Cohen, Weisman & Vazquez, 1988).

Psychological considerations must also be taken into account as HIV testing efforts are increased among the disenfranchised. Learning of one's antibody status in the face of poor health care access, lack of health insurance and lowered levels of self-esteem due to prejudice may result in mental health difficulties leading to and including suicidal risks. And many experience the need to confront their own internalized AIDSism, which is built on fears of homo-sexuality, addicts, death and contagion (Cohen, 1989).

An AIDS related crisis of hopelessness, helplessness, and despair can lead to angry acting out sexually or increased IV drug use in some PAAs and HIV+ individuals as they confront–or avoid con-fronting–an impending death. They must be assisted in completing "unfinished business" with loved ones. Providers must attempt the difficult task of empowering the unemployed or underemployed to write a "will." Clients need not provide financially for their fami-lies, but rather provide plans of care for their children or define how and where they wish to die.

Counselors are reminded that for some the thought of suicide may be the only feeling of control they have over their destiny, and that it can be either consciously or unconsciously promoted by significant others who are themselves unable to accept AIDS (Co-hen, 1990). Care should also be taken to avoid medicating away the very coping skills that some PAAs develop, such as anger and sadness, that may keep them alive and are realistic feelings to have in the face of multiple losses. For disenfranchised people of color, learning to channel these feelings productively through constructive confrontation in the service of health, similar to the technique prac-ticed by ACT-UP, may be helpful.

Biopsychosocial competent health approaches for AIDS-affected people of color would attend to the strengths inherent in cultural views such as the reported holistic view of mental and physical health that some ethnic groups have. Traditional Chinese medicine with its emphasis on prevention, exploration of the underlying causes of illness and reliance on non-invasive treatment approaches (Kinzey, 1991) offers a sensitive intervention to AIDS care which already has been emulated by progressive health providers in the U.S. For example, multi-cultural social workers often consider referral to acupuncturists given Chinese medicine's view of HIV infection as a manageable chronic illness requiring regular surveil-lance to prevent progression and attention to attitudinal factors in maintenance of symptoms (AIDS Action Committee, 1990).

Indeed, it may be that the United States and other western health care systems can learn much from the respect given to holistic inter-ventions on the global and international level. For example, the

World Health Organization, and the Native American tribal and Chinese governments support traditional medical approaches, practitioners, diagnoses and prescriptions in concert with modern medicine.

Human service workers in general and counselors in particular have an opportunity to empower HIV+ persons of color by recognizing those who are independent, alert and who do not wish to be viewed as dependent, controlled patients. The personhood of HIV+ individuals should be acknowledged by encouraging their participation in decision making (McKusick, 1991); advocating for increased protection of their confidentiality (McKusick, 1991a); teaching them how to make bureaucracies work for them (Smith, 1991); and mobilizing them to negotiate health maintenance strategies, including exercising their right to stop medication or treatment at any time. Given that persons of color are more likely to have been disempowered by previous contacts with medical authority, a proactive stance encouraged and modeled by a worker who positively regards and "teams up" with the patient to develop a support network, teach new assertive communication skills, mediate disputes with other providers, and who honestly allows as much control as possible is highly therapeutic (McKusick, 1991b).

Finally, it should be recognized that even when culturally and racially competent AIDS prevention messages exist there may be some individuals whose lives are so filled with other threats to their survival such as homicide, trauma, accidents or poverty (Bowser, 1990) that they will not be reached. The percent of those so affected is impossible to calculate. However, not knowing their numbers cannot keep us from further developing biopsychosocial and community oriented approaches.

COMMUNITY HEALTH MODEL IS MOST APPROPRIATE

Policymakers, activists, and educators have joined in calling for a holistic, human services health approach (Petrovich, 1987) to AIDS that is often not available in an acute care hospital. The ambulatory AIDS/HIV+ patient is offered care by acute hospitals that is often non-continuous, non-comprehensive, uncoordinated, and unmanaged (Cooke & Brooks, 1991). Inpatient care suffers at the point of discharge into the community because of poor hospital communication and referral networks with community based organizations (CBOs) that might provide services of a primary and secondary nature (Abramson & Kark, 1983). The impact on the consumer is that for the inpatient, short stays became long stays due to difficulty in securing placement and home health care, and for outpatients, care is fragmented and costly both in terms of money and time spent waiting to be seen in overcrowded clinics or, worse yet, emergency rooms.

Thus public hospitals, even those with a long history of serving communities of color, the poor, substance users and PAAs, are striving to develop and expand non-hospital based primary care services (Cooke & Brooks, 1991) and to decrease utilization of their emergency rooms and outpatient clinics. Such efforts have been bolstered by no less an authority than the Robert Wood Johnson Foundation's AIDS Health Services Program, a four year effort to develop community based care systems in 11 cities as proof of their effectiveness in medical and social service delivery to PAAs (Vladeck, 1991).

Cohen (1982) defines community health centers (CHCs) as sites where a designated population receives social and ambulatory health care of a preventive and curative nature. Their raison d'etre and targeted funding led to CHCs being established and strategically placed in racially, ethnically, and language diverse communities. Key to the philosophy of these centers is a coordinated, multidisciplinary, mobile, health promoting and managed care delivery of service. Historically, despite being fiscally threatened, CHCs have been successful in providing high quality, low cost prevention and treatment services to the medically underserved, e.g., 70% of CHC patients are people of color (National Association of Community Health Centers, 1990).

In the context of AIDS and communities of color, CHCs are better prepared to thoroughly address HIV/AIDS concerns because of their emphasis on the health of the community as a whole and on the groups which compose it (Abramson & Kark, 1983). For example, maternal child health is a cornerstone of CHC services, and for women and children, AIDS is a disease primarily of communities of color (Harris & Hall, 1988).

In the U.S.A., CHCs historically have actively recruited and employed neighborhood residents, professionals of color and women who act as multi-cultural social change agents and role models in economically and socially distressed communities. Thus, multi-cultural social workers with their proven expertise in communication and administration skills are at the forefront in further development of community health models for AIDS service delivery. CHCs are preferred over other possible community health models such as off-site hospital satellite or extension clinics because of their greater programmatic and fiscal autonomy and accountability to community boards. This last point is a very important one for communities of color as many satellite or extension clinics have at best only an "advisory community body" and at worst, none at all. The CHC has a greater potential to thus reflect the needs of community members who have experienced the negative and positive impact of culture, ethnicity, race, class and gender on their collective and individual health.

INTERVENTIONS

The U.S. health system has failed to provide people of color with access to socio-politically competent and community based AIDS programs. However, interventions can be made more responsive to the ecostructural realities of specific groups. In these interventions, efforts should always be made both to work with, not against, the culture and to draw on the collective strengths of healing approaches that exist in various communities. Moreover, the class competence of AIDS intervention programs can be strengthened by employing local residents as community health workers.

Prevention strategies include developing street or block-based AIDS education programs for low-income women (Drucker, 1990) as they are the diffusers of health knowledge to other adults and children (Hoffman et al., 1991). Folk healers can also be recruited into transmission reduction campaigns and trained to teach other healers about the risks involved in "bleeding" patients and other practices that create exposure to bodily fluids (Eckholm, 1990). In the realm of treatment, acupuncture can be used to build up the immune system, reduce stress, provide symptom relief (Washburn, Keenan & Nazareno, 1990), and treat "crack"–cocaine dependency (Smith, 1989).

Another strategy involves using the performing arts to communicate educational and preventive information. For example, once screened by community representatives, AIDS videos can be used in community health centers as well as hospital waiting and emergency rooms, followed by discussion and debate (Coalition of Hispanic Health and Human Services Organizations, 1989). Peer leaders can be trained to produce interactive theater workshops, newsletters, *Novelas* (Latino soap operas) and videotapes of the workshops, as well as to canvass neighborhood residents (Hispanic Office of Planning and Evaluation, 1991).

Multi-cultural responsive AIDS research can begin by including more people of color in AIDS trials. Thus, research can be done in areas that are relevant to the needs and interests of these communities. This might include developing less obtrusive vaginal condoms that females might use without having to depend on male cooperation (Woodward, 1990) and testing the effects of "natural" remedies like aloe vera, Vitamins C and E, Zinc, garlic, artemisia annua, and acidophilus (AIDS Treatment News, 1986).

Finally, efforts should be made to increase access to community-based settings, which may require deploying AIDS service teams, providers, and child care services from hospital clinics to off-site health centers or decentralized CBOs (Drucker, 1990). Such programs can be incorporated into both community health centers and other places that are frequented by the target population. Thus, AIDS-focused primary health care services can be provided on-site by drug treatment programs, particularly methadone maintenance programs (Selwyn et al., 1989). Likewise, HIV counseling, screening, and testing can be provided in migrant farm health centers, rural clinics, and occupational health centers. In addition, small ethnic/racial and women's business enterprises–such as gypsy cab/van companies, laundromats, dry cleaning stores, record stores, movie theaters, video arcades, bars, restaurants, *bodegas,* and mom and pop stores–can become centers for distribution of prevention materials.

POLICY INITIATIVES

Any discussion of health care policy and human service delivery models in communities of color should at a minimum consider the social justice impact on the individual, groups and organizations within those communities. This involves an examination of how social institutions, and environmental factors, can be combined into forces that do not further victimize populations that are already politically disenfranchised. Additional factors, such as how a problem is defined, results of evaluation of programs, and community development efforts, should be involved in policy setting and analysis.

Sylvia Witts-Vitale (National Puerto Rican Coalition, 1990) speaks of the hierarchy in the AIDS community that places homeless people of color at the bottom and middle class Caucasian men at the top. Her comments are bolstered by medical experts' claims that the most pressing need is for non-medical residential housing for HIV+/PWA "street people," and by legislative inaction on funding for such programs due to concerns regarding their location (Krajicek, 1990). Needless to say, the homeless, IVDUs and communities of color do not have the lobbying power of the generally affluent Caucasian gay community (Mitchell, 1990; Slack, 1992). Yet, communities of color have critics in the gay Caucasian community who feel that gays of color should organize themselves as Caucasians did, without recognition of the lesser income, greater family responsibilities, substandard education and other day-to-day struggle groups of color are more prone to experience (Mitchell, 1990). For example, the needs of communities of color argue for the creation of a national syphilis and tuberculosis prevention, screening and treatment campaign, as these diseases both are highly concentrated among people of color and increase the likelihood of AIDS transmission and weaken the immune systems of PAAs (Edelson, 1990). Other potentially beneficial initiatives and policies include mandating the inclusion of IVDUs in AIDS research, and requiring that all health care providers receive multicultural training that prepares them to respond to AIDS in a competent manner. In all cases, more money should be allocated for these and other community based initiatives that will improve the delivery of AIDS services to people of color.

POSTSCRIPT

With conservative politicians using AIDS to call for harsher social mores or discriminatory legislation, it is difficult for many people of color not to lean toward conspiracy theories when AIDS policy making occurs. Such theories are a measure of the frustration and anger bred by long-standing racial inequities. Their worst impact is that they might erode the credibility of AIDS education, and make people of color feel even more victimized and powerless. From a public health perspective these theories limit the individuals' possibilities to change behavior or recognize their own risk and responsibility (De Parle, 1990).

For many people of color, AIDS prevention campaigns and HIV tests and treatments are not trusted due to a belief that AIDS is "germ warfare" against "undesirable" populations, that there has been a conspiracy of neglect by governmental agencies and a genocidal intent in encouraging condom use, experimental drug trials and methadone or needle exchange programs (De Parle, 1990). These fears are buttressed by Third World rates of morbidity and mortality among communities of color in areas such as cancer, infant mortality, measles, and tuberculosis (Lee, 1991).

If we as human service professionals are to challenge these perceptions, then we cannot procrastinate in disclosing critical research findings (Hilts, 1991). We must not engage in self-serving debates about national health insurance and we must not develop complex and lengthy grant applications that limit CBO competition (Slack, 1992). Instead we must acknowledge the importance of politics and culture, on the workplace, housing and the economy as we develop AIDS policy and service delivery. We must contribute to the reformation of the current care system by addressing the need for additional community health centers, more primary health care workers and universal access to quality health services. We must be true to our ethical and professional obligations to protect the public and serve the people, for health care is a right not a privilege.

REFERENCES

Abramson, J.H. & Kark, S.L. (1983). Community oriented primary care: Meaning and scope. In E. Connor & F. Mullen (Eds.) *Community Oriented Primary Care: New directions for health services delivery–Conference proceedings.* Washington, D. C.: Institute of Medicine.

AIDS Action Committee. (1990). Acupuncture and HIV. *Wellspring: AIDS Action Committee of Massachusetts Newsletter for People with AIDS/ARC,* August 11.

AIDS Treatment News. (1986). AIDS treatment practitioners present natural therapies. *AIDS Treatment News,* 12, 47.

Bowser, B.P. (1990). AIDS & hidden populations. *MIRA Newsletter,* 4 (1),1-2.

Broyles, G.L. (1991). Confab on clinical trials. *The Drum,* 1, 3-4.

Campos, A.P. (1988). A Puerto Rican perspective to counseling. *Counseling and Treating People of Color,* 1 (1), 2.

Coalition of Hispanic Health and Human Services Organizations. (1989). *AIDS: A guide for Hispanic leadership.* Washington, D.C.: Coalition of Hispanic Health and Human Services Organizations.

Cohen, L.G. (1982). Neighborhood health centers: The promise, the rhetoric and the reality. *Journal of Latin Community Health,* 1 (1), 93-100.

Cohen, M.A. & Weisman, H.W. (1986). A biopsychosocial approach to AIDS. *Psychosomatics,* 27, 245-249.

Cohen, M.A., Weisman, H.W., & Vazquez, C. (1988). The acquired immunodeficiency syndrome: a psychiatric crisis. *New York Medical Quarterly,* 8, 53-58.

Cohen, M.A. (1989). AIDSism: a new form of discrimination. *AMA News,* January 20, 43.

Cohen, M.A.A. (1990). Biopsychosocial approach to the human immunodeficiency virus epidemic. A clinician's primer. *General Hospital Psychiatry,* 12, 98-123.

Cooke, J. & Brooks, P. (1991). *Hospitals and the poor: Strategies for primary care.* New York: United Hospital Fund.

Cotton, D., Feinberg, J., & Finkelstein, D. (1991). Participation of women in a multicenter HIV clinical trials program in the United States. Presented at VII International Conference on AIDS, Florence, Italy, June 18.

Cowley, G., Hager, M., & Marshall, R. (1990). AIDS: The next ten years. *Newsweek,* June 25, 20-27.

De Parle, J. (1990). Talk of government being out to get Blacks falls on more attentive ears. *New York Times,* October 29.

Drucker, E. (1990). AIDS in the war zone: Community survival in New York City. *International Journal of Health Services,* 20 (4), 601-615.

Eckholm, E. (1990). AIDS and folk healing, a Zimbabwe encounter. *New York Times,* October 5.

Edelson, E. (1990). Syphilis rate rose by a third in '80s. *New York Daily News,* September 19.

Harris, S. E. & Hall, J.Y. (1988). The impact of AIDS/HIV infection on maternal and pediatric ambulatory care services in New York City's multi-hospital/ facility system. Presented at 116th Annual Meeting, American Public Health Association, Boston, November 17.

Helms, J.E. (1990). What's in a name change? *Focus: Notes from the Society for the Psychological Study of Ethnic Minority Issues,* 4 (2), 1-2.

Hilts, P.J. (1991). Health agency is urged to improve management of its AIDS research. *New York Times,* March 8.

Hispanic Office of Planning and Evaluation. (1991). LUCES: Shedding the light on AIDS. *Hispanic Office of Planning and Evaluation Perspectives,* Fall, 30-31.

Hoffman, S., Grizer, M., De Brosse, S., McLaughlin, C.A., Williams, N., Fahs, M., & Garibaldi, K. (1991). Evaluating community-based AIDS education program for women of color in "high-risk" communities. Presented at 119th Annual Meeting American Public Health Association, Atlanta, November.

Holmberg, D. (1988). AIDS and the poor: Numbers grow but care still lags. *New York Newsday,* May 22, 3.

Kinzey, D.A. (1991). AIDS in the People's Republic of China: A report on the Sino-American information exchange on management of HIV disease. *Psychology & AIDS Exchange,* 5, 1-3.

Krajicek, D.J. (1990). Funding the fight against AIDS. *Empire State Report,* October, 9-44.

Kolata, G. (1991). In medical research equal opportunity doesn't always apply. *New York Times,* March 10.

Lee, D.A. & Fong, K. (1990). HIV/AIDS and the Asian and Pacific Islander community. *SIECUS Report,* 18 (3), 16-22.

Lee, F.R. (1991). Immunization of children said to lag. Third world rate seen in New York area. *New York Times,* October 16.

Menendez, B.S., Drucker, E., Vermund, S.H., Rivera Castano, R., Perez-Agosto, R.R., Parga, F.J., & Blum, S. (1990). AIDS mortality among Puerto Ricans and other Hispanics in New York City. 1981-1987. *Journal of Acquired Immune Deficiency Syndromes,* 3, 644-648.

Mitchell, A. (1990). AIDS: We are not immune. *EMERGE,* 2 (2), 30-44.

McCartney, T. (1988). Obeah and superstition as variables in Bahamian mental health difficulties. *Counseling and Treating People of Color,* 1 (1), 2.

McKusick, L. (1991). *HIV Frontline No. 1–April.*

McKusick, L. (1991a). *HIV Frontline No. 2–May.*

McKusick, L. (1991b). *HIV Frontline No. 5–November.*

National Association of Community Health Centers. (1990). Access 2000: A plan to provide basic health care to all uninsured Americans. Unpublished Ms: National Association of Community Health Centers.

National Puerto Rican Coalition. (1990). Jose Gonzalez house offers refuge to New York's forgotten people. *National Puerto Rican Coalition Reports,* July-August 3.

Petrovich, J. (1987). *Northeast Hispanic needs: A guide for action. Volume 2.* Washington, D.C.: ASPIRA Institute for Policy Research.

Rendon, M. (1984). Myths and stereotypes in minority groups. *International Journal of Social Psychology,* 30 (4), 297-309.

Rosenthal, E. (1990). Health problems of inner city poor reach crisis point. *New York Times,* December 24.

Rowell, R.M. (1990). Native Americans, stereotypes, and HIV/AIDS: Our continuing struggle for survival. *SIECUS Report,* 18 (3), 9-15.

Salas Rojas, A. (1992). Latinos fight against AIDS. *New York Newsday,* January 14.

Selik, R.M., Castro, K.G., Pappaioanou, M., & Buehler, J.W. (1989). Birthplace and the risk of AIDS among Hispanics in the United States. *American Journal of Public Health,* 78, 1539-1545.

Selwyn, P.A., Feingold, A.R., Iezza, A., Sat Yadeo, M., Colley, J., Torres, R., & Shaw, J.F.M. (1989). Primary care for patients with human immunodeficiency virus (HIV) infection in a methadone maintenance treatment program. *Annals of Internal Medicine,* 110 (9), 761-763.

Slack, J.D. (1992). The public administration of AIDS. *Public Administration Review,* 52 (1), 77-81.

Smith, M. (1991). Problems confronting Blacks. *HIV Frontline,* 2, 5.

Smith, M.O. (1989). Testimony presented to the select committee on narcotics of the U.S. House of Representatives. The Lincoln Hospital Drug Abuse Program, July 25.

Tafoya, T. (1991). Testing for HIV in Native American communities: Special considerations. *HIV Frontline,* 2, 7.

Vladeck, B. (1991). Foreword. *In* S.A.R. Masline. *If we knew then what we know now: Planning for people with AIDS. Paper Series 15.* New York: United Hospital Fund.

Washburn, A.M., Keenan, P.A., & Nazareno, J.P. (1990). Preliminary findings: Study of acupuncture-assisted heroin detoxification. *MIRA Newsletter,* 40 (1), 3-6.

Woodward, C. (1990). AIDS stats bad news for women. *New York Newsday,* July 11, 6.

For Product Safety Concerns and Information please contact our EU
representative GPSR@taylorandfrancis.com Taylor & Francis Verlag GmbH,
Kaufingerstraße 24, 80331 München, Germany

Batch number: 08153776

Printed by Printforce, the Netherlands